The Emotional Survival Guide for Caregivers

Looking After Yourself and Your Family While Helping an Aging Parent

BARRY J. JACOBS, PsyD

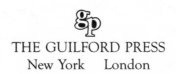

THE GUILFORD PRESS
New York   London

© 2006 The Guilford Press
A Division of Guilford Publications, Inc.
72 Spring Street, New York, NY 10012
www.guilford.com

The information in this volume is not intended as a substitute for
consultation with healthcare professionals. Each individual's health
concerns should be evaluated by a qualified professional.

Printed in the United States of America

This book is printed on acid-free paper.

Last digit is print number: 9   8   7   6   5   4   3   2   1

Library of Congress Cataloging-in-Publication Data

Jacobs, Barry J.
  The emotional survival guide for caregivers : looking after yourself and your
family while helping an aging parent / Barry J. Jacobs.
     p. cm.
  Includes index.
  ISBN-10 1-59385-295-9   ISBN-13 978-1-59385-295-5 (hardcover: alk paper)
  ISBN-10 1-57230-729-3   ISBN-13 978-1-57230-729-2 (paperback: alk paper)
  1. Aging parents—Care.   2. Caregivers—Psychology.   3. Adult children
of aging parents—Family relationships. I. Title.
  HQ1063.6.J33 2006
  649.8084'6—dc22   2005034070

Pages 1–2 of the Prologue are adapted from Jacobs (1998). In Sickness & Health:
Termites. *Families, Systems, & Health, 16*(3), 323–324. Copyright 1998 by the
Educational Publishing Foundation by assignment to the American Psychological
Association. Adapted by permission.

Question and answer sections at the end of most chapters are adapted from Jacobs
(2002, 2003, 2005). What Can I Do? In *Take Care!: Self-Care for the Family Caregiver*,
Vols. 1–4 for 2002 and 2003; Vols. 1–2 for 2005. Copyright 2002, 2003, 2005 by the
National Family Caregivers Association. Adapted by permission.

About the Author

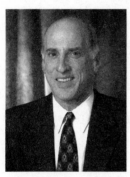 **Barry J. Jacobs, PsyD,** works with couples and families coping with serious health problems. He has faculty appointments at Temple University, the University of Pennsylvania, and Widener University, and is the Director of Behavioral Sciences for the Crozer-Keystone Family Medicine Residency Program in Springfield, Pennsylvania. He is also a widely published journalist who has written extensively for *The Village Voice* and other publications. Currently, he writes an advice column for *Take Care!*, the quarterly newsletter of the National Family Caregivers Association, edits the "In Sickness & Health" column for the journal *Families, Systems & Health,* and maintains a website for the public at www.emotionalsurvivalguide.com. He lives with his wife and their two children in Swarthmore, Pennsylvania.

Contents

Acknowledgments

From the patients' family members I first met in a rehabilitation unit almost 20 years ago to the ones I met last week in the family medicine center where I now work, from those I saw only once to those I've seen dozens of times over many years, I've learned a tremendous amount from the caregivers with whom I've worked. They've taught me there's a broad range of normal reactions, including ambivalence, to a loved one's serious illness. By sharing with me their sensitivity and pluck, anguish and resilience, they've demonstrated how to be human and yet go on through often excruciating family circumstances. More than anyone else, they supplied insights that are the core of this book. I'm very grateful for my time with them.

Many other people have helped me along the way. Through his struggles with cancer, my father never stopped showing that he loved me, my brother, and my mother. During his illness and afterward, my mother made many difficult sacrifices to keep our family going. My brother has always been my partner in using humor to cope, even in the face of our family's medical ordeal. I thank them all.

I've been blessed with many terrific mentors and colleagues. At Brown University, the late Roger Henkle taught me the value of storytelling; Robert Jay taught me to trust experience as a basis for knowledge. At the Institute for Graduate Clinical Psychology of Widener University, supervising psychologists Hugh Carberry and Leighton Whitaker gave me an appreciation for the therapeutic value of sadness.

In my previous position as a psychologist at Bryn Mawr Rehab, psychologists Ann Marie McLaughlin and Jim Jaep and neurologist David Long helped me understand the ways that families deal with traumatic brain injuries and other neurological disorders. In my current job at the Crozer-Keystone Family Medicine Residency Program, I've been fortunate to receive the support and encouragement of Mitchell Kaminski, William Warning, David Berkson, our fellow faculty members, and a great staff, and have also enjoyed the enthusiasm of dozens of past and present family medicine residents. Colleague Peter Warrington, a family physician and geriatrician who also completed a residency in obstetrics/gynecology, did a meticulous job going over the medical details in this book.

University of Rochester psychologist and family therapist Susan McDaniel deserves special thanks for spearheading the fields of medical family therapy and collaborative family healthcare and for providing me encouragement and opportunity to share my own ideas; from 1995 onward, she's allowed me to write, and later edit, the "In Sickness & Health" column in the journal she coedits with family physician Thomas Campbell, *Families, Systems, & Health*. Suzanne Mintz, cofounder of the National Family Caregivers Association, gives me the privilege of writing the "What Can I Do?" advice column for *Take Care!*, the quarterly newsletter of her organization; Sandy Rogers, the newsletter editor, is generous with her support, guidance, and good cheer. To my close friend and colleague David Seaburn, with whom I share interests in families and writing, I owe gratitude for plenty of insights and laughs.

The family caregiving field has many skilled leaders. I've already mentioned Suzanne Mintz of the National Family Caregivers Association, one of the most creative and determined people I've ever met. Carol Levine of the United Hospital Fund of New York City, a visionary for creating and funding new caregiver support programs, has been an inspiring figure of grace, intelligence, and wry humor. The Rosalynn Carter Institute for Caregiving has long been a leader in caregiver research and raising public awareness; it was an honor for me to participate on its cancer and caregiving national expert panel. The Well Spouse Association has afforded me several opportunities to present to its members and partake of its particular high-spirited and often hilarious camaraderie.

I thank Guilford Publications for the chance to write this book. Kitty Moore helped me formulate the original vision. Sarah Lavender Smith challenged me often with practical questions that helped me ground my thinking. My main editor, Christine Benton, provided me with more empathy, support, and encouragement than I've received from practically anyone else in my life. I've told her she should be a psychologist. (Honestly, I mean that in a good way.) It has been pure joy working closely with her.

My greatest thanks, though, go to my family. My children, Monica and Aaron, are two good people with spunk and curiosity. My wife, Julie Mayer, has been an incisive reader of books and people and my greatest friend. For their love and forbearance, I dedicate this book to them.

Prologue

When I was 13, my father's law practice had finally taken off and my family was able to afford its first home after years of high-rise apartment dwelling. It was a modest prewar ranch house in Queens, New York, with three bedrooms and an addition—a former screened-in porch turned into a walnut-paneled den—surrounded by rhododendrons, azaleas, and a towering white oak. The den was designated as my father's domain as a reward for years of hard toil. He set up his leather recliner and hardcover books there and was always given the choice of channel on the Zenith 19-inch color TV. He'd come home late, eat quickly, and retire to his den to put his feet up after his day of battling in court.

It was in that room one night, 18 months after we'd moved in, that our simple normal life came to an end. My father turned to a visiting friend, opened his mouth, and emitted gibberish. The look of shock on his face indicated that he realized he'd made no sense. He tried speaking again, and again the sounds came out in a mixed-up salad that had pieces of English words but no discernible meaning. With that moment, he'd lost the power of intelligible speech. In the months that followed, he partially lost the abilities to see and to balance himself. It was just before the advent of CT scans, and the doctors could only guess that a malignant cell growth was raging in his brain. I was too young to understand much, but I clearly sensed my mother's terror. My father, meanwhile, was alternately mum and angry. We all pinned our hopes on the drastic course of chemotherapy he was to undergo.

A few weeks after he began the chemotherapy, my mother called an exterminator because she'd seen flying ants outside our home and was afraid they were termites. Several men came with hoses and a big drill and pumped poison into a series of holes dug into the ground around the perimeter of the house. Several days later, my mother, father, 11-year-old brother, and I were sitting in the den after dinner when suddenly I noticed that the floor was covered with tens of thousands of wriggling black insect bodies. The termites, driven into the house's interior by the poison, were swarming up through the wooden threshold that connected the den addition to the rest of the house. I can still see their translucent wings twitching, hear their low buzz, and feel the crunch of their bodies as I stood up and crossed the room. I was gagging with horror even as I ran to the front hall closet to get the vacuum cleaner. In that instant when our house was being invaded by these grotesque bugs, my young mind grasped that they were like the cancer cells that had infiltrated our lives. My mother and I spent an hour silently vacuuming and sweeping them up while my brother sat stock-still in fear and my father stumbled about the room, unable to help us because he didn't have the eyesight to distinguish the shiny black bodies all over the patterned carpet.

Afterward, we said nothing to each other about the termites but were all spooked. I remember thinking the swarm was a portent that my father's cancer cells would still grow uncontrollably, evading whatever poisons the doctors used. Five months later, he was dead.

It was my first lesson in how serious illness affects not just individuals but their devoted family members. We tried our best to give care to my dad. But the cancer was like some infestation, devouring the economic, emotional, and spiritual foundations of our lives and forever weakening the structure of our family. I did not know it at the time, but the event also became the impetus for my entire professional career and for this book—to help members of other caregiving families avoid the damage that we suffered.

The economic damage was most immediately evident. After a steady rise in prosperity, it was jarring to drop a few levels. Once my father became sick, he shuffled the legal papers on his desk in the den and even went downtown to his office a couple of times, but these were merely hopeful gestures; he was never able to really work again. To make up for the shortfall from his dwindling income, my mother took a full-time job as a bookkeeper that kept her out of the house for long hours. Like all economic decisions, it had relationship fallout. My father's parents wanted her at home caring for their son, regardless of how little money we had. Although my 83-year-old grandfather sat in the den with my dad watching TV while we were at work or school, he'd leave brusquely to catch the subway as soon as we returned. My grandmother was not nearly so diplomatic and lambasted my mother repeatedly in heated phone calls. A schism between my grandparents and mother had emerged. If my father minded that his wife was working or his parents were worked up, he was never able to say.

After he passed into a coma and died, further economic changes increased the emotional damage. My mother took a second job teaching college math in the evenings. I started working weekends in my uncle's carpet cleaning business. Between her work and mine, her forays into dating and my hanging out with fellow teens, I hardly ever saw her. It was like I'd lost two parents. We were all so busy that no one was talking about what we were feeling. The sadness that hovered around us never got processed between us and so remained a constant presence. Then, 2 years later, my mother brought home the man who was going to be her new husband. The focus then shifted to forming a new family, and any chance was lost for my brother, mother, and me to clear the air of all that had happened before. My father's parents, meanwhile, had long since avoided their sad feelings by using my mom as a scapegoat. They cut off all contact with her as soon as my father was buried, blaming her for neglecting him during his decline. My brother and I continued seeing them periodically, but our relationship with them was now strained. The losses stemming from the illness kept mounting.

Calamitous loss can have two opposing effects. It can strengthen one's grip on the present, making sensations and relationships all the more precious for fear they'll also be lost; this is hyperawareness of the "make every day count" and "smell the roses" variety. Or it can render one numb to current circumstances as if they are already as good as gone; this was the spiritual damage I suffered. I was coming into a doubting age even before my father became ill. Watching the slow decimation of this good man was hard to comprehend except as evidence that the world didn't make sense. His death, despite modern medicine and intensely felt prayers, sealed it for me: There was no God watching out for us, no just ending. There were only work duties and family rifts and unvocalized despair.

The path out of this for me was circuitous. At college, I had a tendency to befriend others who had experienced family illnesses and tragedies. After graduation, I became a magazine journalist drawn to writing stories about how people coped with traumatic changes. In hindsight, it's clear I was groping for a handle on my own experience. But even when I left journalism for a doctoral program in clinical psychology with the vague aspiration of helping people, I was little aware I'd been seeking ways to help myself.

And then during my third year in the psychology program, nearly 15 years after my father's death, a chance event changed my life. I needed to find a clinical practicum site reachable by public transportation, and the only one available was the physical medicine rehabilitation unit of a local hospital. I didn't even know what rehab was. But from the first week I arrived there to counsel patients and family members dealing with strokes, amputations, head injuries, and brain cancer, I felt like I was finally turning full attention to a neglected part of myself. Their struggles with fear and uncertainty were replays of my family's; their shock and grief echoed within me. I found that I could empathize instantly with their reactions and effortlessly knew the right words to comfort them. The effect was revelatory. It was as if an avenue had opened before me that was not just going to be my career path but a direct connection between the troubling thoughts and feelings of my past and a redemptive mission for the future. The mission was that of many wounded healers: Lead others safely over dangerous roads where I myself once crashed. I would never be able to quell all the destructive forces that were part of any passage through illness; I could only try to teach family members the survival skills for continuing to move forward until they reached safer ground and a new, more hopeful place.

In the 20 years since, there has continued to be interplay between my personal history and my passion for helping caregiving families. While I guard against superimposing my troubles on their traumas (I only rarely have shared my story), I bring ingrained beliefs from my early experiences to my clinical work. Because I was so affected by my father's sickness and death, I state emphatically to my clients that serious illness occurs to families, not just individuals. When a loved one is sick, it sends waves of emotion throughout the extended family system, altering the landscape of relationships. Because my family was swamped by this wake, I add just as emphatically that how well caregivers deal with a loved one's disability will shape the ways they function for years to come. The resentments created when relatives argue over caregiving or abandon each other have lasting power. So do the bonds forged when family members caregive together harmoniously. The bratty little sister you always considered selfish seems more loving and formidable after sharing responsibility for an ailing parent with you. The difficult spouse you long thought distant rises in your esteem by rallying to the cause of providing ongoing care.

But the strongest bias I share is that family members need to communicate with one another about their feelings and thoughts to strategize handling the illness in order to sustain the family. In my experience, not talking together only makes caregiving efforts disjointed, intensifies feelings of helplessness, and undermines all semblance of family coherence. It's like a group of creative cooks in a kitchen who, never talking with one another about a menu, work feverishly with pots and skillets and all make the same dish—or make a wild assortment of dishes that won't taste good together. Or it's like a basketball team without set plays or verbal signals whose players keep tripping over one another's sneakers and throwing the ball out of bounds.

Just as my personal experiences have affected my clinical judgment, my clinical experience colors how I perceive my history. When I sit with the distraught wife of a man with cancer, I feel keenly her sense of panic and despair as I tap into my own reservoir of emotions stemming from my family's cancer crisis. Connecting the clinical moment with the old feelings leads me to compare the woman's reaction with that of my mother. Did she go through the same tumult when my father was sick, I wonder, without my having appreciated it at the time? As a result of this associative chain, I hear the woman more intently while feeling a growing empathy for my mom. When I meet angry, aged parents who decry the aloofness of the husband of their stroke-stricken daughter, I gain respect for the righteous loyalty of my grandparents in a way that wasn't possible when they were attacking Mom. Sharing in these families' lives, I relive and learn about my own family's ordeal. For that privilege, I feel grateful every day.

I've written this book to help family members—in particular, adult children of ill, aging parents, because you are the biggest group of family caregivers today—identify means of effectively mustering their energies to help a seriously ill loved one while also taking preventive steps to limit caregiving's debilitating effects on the family as a whole. It's about doing the right thing for someone in need without risking creating other family problems, in either the near or long term. It's about practicing love and loyalty in the smartest, most flexible fashion by being aware of the costs of the commitments you make but also the potential rewards of sacrificing for higher aims. First-time caregivers will find a useful road map of the challenges to be confronted at each stage of the journey. You'll be able to dip into specific chapters to read about a variety of families at similar junctures learning their own diverse ways for succeeding. Experienced caregivers will gain greater insight into the interpersonal interactions between patients and relatives, between relatives and professionals, and among the range of individuals—hot-headed to easygoing, stoic to ebullient—that make up the cast of characters of any family tested over the course of a serious illness. You'll be able to recognize most of your own emotional reactions as normal and empathize more surely with others' unique responses.

The book is organized around the story of a caregiving family and its cancer-riddled matriarch. It isn't based on any one family from my personal or professional experience. Rather, it's a conglomeration of many families and intended to represent an ordinary loving clan that finds itself fighting serious illness. I've taken a middle path with the depictions of the patient and family members. No one here is exemplary; they're neither heroes nor villains. The sisters you'll meet aren't going to be likable to everyone. They make plenty of mistakes and can go at each other when under stress. I think they're typical caregivers. By the same token, I haven't depicted exemplary healthcare professionals but ones whose skills and manners I'd regard as average. They're typical people too, with good and bad attributes, doing the best they can in an extremely flawed healthcare system. In short, they're very human. They suffer in this rendering to some degree from the fact that what you'll see of them is through the eyes of the patient and caregivers.

An introductory chapter describes the family at the initial stage of the matriarch's diagnosis. It offers research findings and clinical anecdotes to explore the impact of serious illness on families and of family caregiving on the course of a loved one's disease. It also introduces two ideas that are mainstays for the rest of the book: First, the relationships among well and ill family members and healthcare providers generally determine whether caregiving can be sustained over time. Second, however satisfying or helpful these relationships are will be shaped to a great degree by how successfully or poorly family members grapple with seven basic psychological tasks.

These tasks—defining commitments, utilizing support, handling sacrifice, weighing hope and acceptance, fostering awareness and flexibility, protecting intimacy, and sustaining the spirit—are outlined in the seven ensuing chapters. Each chapter follows our caregiving family through time as they cope with medical treatments, sibling arguments, marital spats, misunderstandings with the treating professionals, and the vicissitudes of the disease. At the end of Chapters 1 through 9, there's a section of questions and answers that explore different facets of the caregiving task at hand and offer specific tips and strategies for success. Most of these "Q&As" were originally published in earlier versions in the "What Can I Do?" advice column that I wrote for *Take Care!*, the quarterly newsletter of the National Family Caregivers Association (NFCA), and stem from queries submitted by caregivers from around the country. The Epilogue completes the family's story while also outlining common challenges for relatives once the caregiving work is done. A Resources section at the end of the volume lists a variety of organizations, publications, and websites that offer help for patients and caregiving families about caregiving in general or specific life-altering diseases.

My hope is to impart to caregivers the skills needed to fare as well as possible during and after the serious illness of an aging parent or other loved one. Family life can be upended by prolonged caregiving as surely as persistent termites bore through wood. But by knowing how to recognize the early signs of caregiver fatigue and taking concerted action to support all family members, our families can become stronger, not weaker, through the caregiving experience, deriving greater regard for each member and a deepened love.

CHAPTER ONE

———◯◯———

First Days

At night, after the patients are tucked tightly into their beds, there's a hush in the hospital hallways, and you can hear bad news coming a long way off. A tousled young doctor, rounding on his hospitalized patients after completing his office appointments, charges down the corridor with loafers squeaking on the polished linoleum floor. He stops at the nurse's station, double-checks what he'd been told on the phone by skimming a note in a chart, and then ducks into the room of an 80-year-old woman. Despite the late hour, her two middle-aged daughters are still restlessly perched on plastic chairs by their mother's bedside, dejectedly watching the curled-up woman sleeping. The doctor waves at them to join him in the hall. "As you know," he says breathlessly, "when you brought your mother to the emergency room yesterday for severe back pain, a transvaginal ultrasound found a mass on her right ovary and she was admitted to the hospital for more tests. The results of the laparoscopy conducted today to take tissue samples of that mass aren't good." Pausing, he gives each of them a sympathetic look before stating quietly, "You mother has ovarian cancer. It's a Grade 2, or moderately aggressive, tumor. Probably spread beyond the ovaries. She'll definitely need more surgery." He pauses again and declares, "I'll do all I can to arrange the best care for her. Do you have any questions?" They stare back at him in shock and shake their heads. He then excuses himself and takes off down the hall, white lab coat trailing behind him like a fleeing specter.

The daughters stand there stunned. One gapes, the other cries. They clutch each other's thick hands and say nothing. Years from now, they'll recall the moment as the demarcation point between what they had been—a normal family with an aging but vivacious mother—and what they are to become: an injured, grieving family. Serious illness always arrives with a shock as if a ship, having long drifted on slow currents or glided through open waters, runs up suddenly on unseen rocks. Even among families that face crises with determined upbeatness, there's an initial shudder of fear as the structure of their lives totters. Even family members of a fatalistic bent, who constantly peer ahead for the next bad thing to come, are thrown backwards by the jolt. Even in families in which a parent's age should prepare the daughters for some medical event, a doctor's pronouncement of illness rattles everyday routines with a rumbling crash.

The daughters lean heavily on the railing that lines the hallway wall and slowly begin talking in the low whispers of girls sharing secrets out of Mother's earshot. Though they're both in their fifties, one is 5 years older than the other, and under the moment's duress they revert to the patterned behaviors of big and little sisters. "We've got a lot of things to do. We've got to think things through," the older one says in a pressured tone. The younger one gazes at her expectantly. But the initial shock has given way to only uncertainty for them. What did the doctor mean exactly? they ask themselves. How bad is it really? Did he rush away out of haste or fear of telling them too much and painting too bleak a picture? This is followed by a set of more immediate questions: Are we supposed to tell our mother the test results? Or should we let the doctor tell her tomorrow and then make believe we hadn't known? Their father had died of cancer; won't that make it harder for Mother to handle her diagnosis? And what if it's wrong—should they get a second opinion before saying anything to their mother? And then a third set of pressing questions occurs to them: How can we leave her tonight knowing she has cancer? But what would our husbands think if we don't come home? Are we daughters first or wives?

They hear a couple of nursing aides laughing near the unit secretary's desk. The hallway is otherwise a quiet, lonesome place. The older sister goes into her mother's room momentarily and then comes out again and begins pacing slowly. The younger sister watches her and nervously licks her glossed lips. In all other life crises, they'd look to their mother for guidance. Now, following the doctor's whirlwind visit, that's no longer possible. They're already feeling the loss of the mother they've known.

In antiseptic institutions and offices, during anxious hours of night and day, scenes like this play out. For physicians, they are challenging problems for which biomedicine prescribes evidence-based treatment paths. In a case of cancer, the doctors will consider the type of tumor, the organ in which it's located, and whether an older patient is hardy enough to withstand the arsenal of possible treatments—surgery, chemotherapy, and radiation. But for most people blindsided by a diagnosis, the news occurs against a backdrop of personal and family histories and evokes feelings and associations that have little to do with organic pathology. It's not just that they don't understand the science behind their life-threatening disease. It's that the threat brings those lives into sharper focus. Their memories and dreams, now more vulnerable, seem suddenly more vivid to them. Their relationships with family and friends, revealed as fragile, seem more crucial.

In the morning, when the mother wakes up, she's greeted by her physician, looking studiedly somber, rounding again before his office hours. She glances at her bleary-eyed daughters now slouched in the plastic chairs as if they'd spent the night in them. (They actually went home at their husbands' requests but made sure they returned early so they could be present when the doctor delivered the news.) When the doctor clears his throat and announces in a low voice that her tumor is ovarian cancer, the mother stiffens and then sighs. He goes on to try to explain the specialists he's contacted and the surgery she'll need—at the least, to remove her right ovary—but she's already too preoccupied to hear much of what he says. In those first moments, myriad questions pass through her mind: How much of me will they cut out? Will the pain be bad? Who will take me to the doctor's office? Who will clean my apartment if I get too weak? The physician glances uneasily at her daughters, who nod back slightly. Then he mumbles goodbye to the older woman before making a quick exit again. She's staring toward the window and doesn't answer him.

Over the next hour, the mother and daughters converse sporadically, with long pauses. Her roommate has already turned on her TV, and the cheery tones of the commercials make a surreal background for their gloomy thoughts. The breakfast tray comes, but the mother hardly touches it. She expresses her thoughts in a gruff, even voice that her daughters know she's always used to try to cover all fears. She looks at them hard with her dull blue eyes several times as if trying to gauge whether she can fully depend on them. The makeup on their tired faces is askew, but they appear attentive and concerned. The thought occurs to her that she'll ask no more of them than what she once gave them freely and feels she deserves now—setting aside their busy lives for a while to give her their undivided attention, just as she did, as their mother, for them and, as a wife, for her dying husband.

As the day wears on and her shock begins to fade, the wild multiplication of cells within her still receives little of her thought. Instead, she worries about whether she'll be well enough to make Thanksgiving dinner for the extended family and whether her sons-in-law will resent that her need for care will deprive them of their wives' time. Lying still in bed with her wrinkled face sagging and her silver hair flattened and mussed, she sifts through her past, recalling what it was like for her when she was a child and stared at haggard old people hollowed out by cancer. She wonders what her grandchildren and great-grandchildren will be thinking while watching her in the coming months. She ponders her late husband's choices in his fight against the dread disease, remembering the graciousness with which he faced his death. She feels fresh grief that he can't be there at her side to help her now.

In those moments during that morning when the daughters feel their mother's eyes upon them, they each experience a surge of compassion and protectiveness toward her but also a mild discomfiting shame. Each of them senses intuitively that the serious illness of a loved one brings a kind of reckoning for every family member. Close relatives, especially, feel the press of the tribe's prime rule: Be there in the hour of need. How family members respond to the call to be at the hospital, provide money, or give up their jobs to take a sick parent into their home becomes a measure of their loyalty and love. Though no request has yet been made nor arrangements discussed, the daughters are already aware their mother is taking note of whether they meet or turn away from her plaintive gaze. She'll surely judge them, they figure, for what they do or don't do for her throughout her illness.

The conversation lags, the TV drones, and the lunch tray arrives without fanfare. The daughters notice that their eyes seek out each other whenever they awkwardly sidle between the bed and the tinted window in their half of the tiny room. This is due partly to the unspoken commiseration and camaraderie between them. They look at each other with sad but knowing expressions as if to say "We thought it would be hard if it ever came to this, and it is; we're in this fix together now." But their looks take on a wide-eyed cast at times as if a question hangs in the air for which they need reassurance from each other: Are we really in this together?

What does it mean to be a family caregiver? In some instances, it may initially entail doing a few chores for an aging relative who can no longer take care of her home entirely on her own. As that loved one continues to age, you may be expected to incrementally do more and more for her over time. In other cases, being a caregiver means having to provide 24-hour total care to someone who's been suddenly stricken with a serious illness that has disabled him utterly. In nearly every instance of family caregiving, siblings and other relatives have to negotiate means of tending to their loved one while dividing the labor in a way that feels fair and equitable to everyone involved. Even in the most trusting, committed, and communicative families, there's always some question about who will come through and for how long—not just during the initial crisis but in the months, and possibly years, that follow, when care continues to be needed. When family members don't come through for one another, let alone for the patient, the resulting anger runs deep. Like shared memories of failures to give wedding presents or atrocious behavior at funerals, they recall the disparities of caregiving effort for decades. The hard feelings can harm family relationships beyond repair.

These sisters have always managed whatever conflicts arose between them and were able to cooperate well during their father's decline 10 years before. And yet, more jarring than the crackle of the hospital's paging system, doubts intrude on their thoughts now. The younger one knows her older sister's husband has been set on doing some traveling. Will her sister feel pressure, she wonders, to leave town and Mom? But the younger sister also knows her older sister's inclination to take over situations, and she doesn't want her to grab the glory of doing the bulk of the caregiving. The older one realizes her younger sister has a new grandchild she hoped to baby-sit. Will she sit with their mother as well? The older sister also has long been critical of her younger sibling's passive tendency to let others take the lead. Everything they know of each other's lives—their temperaments, circumstances, and entrenched habits—becomes one of many variables to be weighed in an attempt to discern their caregiving future together.

Here's where the undercurrent of shame comes in. For all their concern about the other's willingness to give care, these daughters are ambivalent about the sacrifices they feel obliged to make. They do want to help their mother live as long as possible with comfort and dignity; they promised their father before he died they would. But they've reached the point in their own full lives where their children and grandchildren need their help while their husbands want them to slow down. No one in the family will openly begrudge them the time they give their mother. But the daughters will feel pressure nonetheless to be just as good grandmothers and wives. They also have jobs. Tending Mom will stretch them thin.

> Many people add shame to the burden of worry, sadness, anger, and dread over a family member diagnosed with a serious illness as they struggle with ambivalence toward the caregiving task that looms ahead. But it's only natural to feel overwhelmed by the prospect of adding caregiving to an already full plate. Ambivalence toward caregiving should be considered a normal, expectable reaction that doesn't invalidate your love or devotion to your ill family member. It's neither necessary nor helpful to feel ashamed.

They little relish caregiving her for other reasons, too. Their mother was always a take-charge lady who guided them firmly. They know she deserves the benefit of their strength now, but they're leery of flipping the mother–child roles and usurping her power. Telling her which pills to take, when to go to bed, what to tell her doctors—it would all be so presumptuous of them. Who are they to compound the injury of cancer with the insult of condescension? The mere possibility that taking charge themselves might detract from who she's been fills them with guilt.

There's also no guarantee that, once they rearrange their lives to meet her needs, it will end anytime soon. Their father may have succumbed relatively quickly, but they know their tough mother will fight longer. The weeks of driving her may stretch into months, the months of comforting her drag into years. If her cancer progresses and she becomes disabled, they'll have to do even more. Lift her? Change her soiled clothes? Anything's possible. At what point would they get sick of it? When would they start feeling resentful? Perhaps they'd even pray for her death one day. It seems inconceivable now, but they've heard of other daughters who long provided hands-on care and became just that desperate for relief.

The afternoon drags on interminably. Their mother tries to nap but is unable to. She then tells the older daughter to make several phone calls for her and directs the younger one to track down her nurse to fetch an extra blanket. The sisters are glad for something constructive to do, although they inwardly recoil in the instant their mother orders them about. While it's normal for family caregivers to harbor negative sentiments, the daughters feel abashed by these feelings. They try to squelch them by refocusing on Mom's needs, straightening her bed, fussing with her hair. Some part of them wants to escape home to their waiting spouses. But they feel compelled to stay so that she's not alone with her worries for too long. It strains them to sit idly for hours, watching her in anguish. But they're both cognizant that, because she has a life-threatening disease, every remaining moment with her is time they should cherish. This is only day 1 of caregiving, and the daughters already feel emotionally and physically spent. They fear their mother will need them for days ahead as far as they can see.

Like most family members, these daughters are struggling with the many possible meanings of sacrifice. For some caregivers, giving their lives over to caring for a loved one will gratify them as the most significant, ennobling endeavor they've ever undertaken. Think of Susan Sarandon as the mother in the movie *Lorenzo's Oil* who relinquishes her work, friendships, and nearly her marriage to seek a cure for her son's terminal congenital condition. The mission of saving him becomes the moving force of her being. Other caregivers experience the sacrifices as a form of entrapment or exploitation. Consider Edith Wharton's novella *Ethan Frome*, in which the careworn husband is repulsed by his griping, pain-addled wife and seeks love outside his marriage. By escaping her, he's trying to transform the embittered and lifeless self that caregiving has rendered him.

These dramatic depictions are the extreme poles of a broad spectrum. Few of the close relatives caught up in caring for an ill parent, spouse, or child are as obsessively devoted as a Susan Sarandon or as piteously downtrodden as an Ethan Frome. Caregiving provokes a wide range of emotional reactions to a complicated life choice involving personal sacrifices to yield family benefit. Most caregivers are likely to experience a mix of emotions about what they do, depending on whether they are reflecting on their lot at any specific instant as individual beings or beholden family members. You may feel proud and angry simultaneously. You may feel angry about being burdened, then feel guilty for having felt anger, and then become angry again for having been made to feel guilty. The combinations are infinite and exhausting. You may find that the tension accompanying your conflicted emotions is a cause of much duress.

In their middle-aged years these sisters have probably known many good people who have taken care of ill loved ones. They may see others' efforts as proof that families have always taken care of their own— that duty wins out over personal excuses and doubts, over work and money, even over all pursuit of happiness. As a consequence, they're likely to castigate themselves for their misgivings and try to shunt them aside. That, however, would do them an injustice. Caregiving has always been hard, no matter how valiantly and heartily some family members have embraced it. As a series of daunting logistical and emotional challenges, it's only becoming more arduous nowadays. For these daughters are embarking on the caregiving journey at a time in the histories of the American medical system and our country's families when there exists a strange paradox: Healthcare professionals have knowledge and technologies at their disposal that make them more self-assured than ever in fighting disease. But the family caregivers of our ill citizens have rarely, if ever, been left so beleaguered.

Several deleterious trends for family members have developed over the past decade. Foremost among them is that increasing numbers of Americans are being asked to set aside some part of their own lives to care for another. According to the National Family Caregivers Association (NFCA), a Washington, DC-based self-help and advocacy group, more than 50 million people in this country provide some care to a relative or friend each year. Of these, about half, or 25 million Americans, the United Hospital Fund of New York City has found, provide ongoing care not just for 1 year but for year after difficult year for seriously ill or disabled family members. In a study by MetLife, the average length of time spent caregiving was 8 years. The largest portion of family caregivers are adult children, like the daughters, who must take care of disabled or demented parents. But increasing percentages also include "well spouses," who tend to ill husbands or wives, as well as parents of chronically ill or disabled children. Regardless of the family role that you play, you're among a steadily growing group of Americans contending with caregiving's stresses. (This phenomenon is hardly exclusive to the United States: The 2001 census in the United Kingdom reported that 5.2 million family members and friends were providing care for a loved one in England and Wales—a full tenth of the population of those nations.)

The causes of this burgeoning phenomenon are many. Some of it is demographic. As the age of the average American continues to rise thanks to generally improved healthcare, the kinds of chronic, debilitating diseases—such as dementia, diabetes, heart disease, and cancer—that ordinarily develop later in life become more prevalent. According to the 2000 report of the National Center for Health Statistics, over 35 million Americans are encumbered in their daily activities by chronic mental health or physical health conditions. More disease means a greater preponderance of symptoms that diminish the day-to-day functioning of older individuals. More infirm and partially disabled older people create the need for increased assistance from others, namely, family members. For example, when a 75-year-old man with high blood pressure and Type II diabetes suffers a minor stroke that slows his reflexes and blurs his vision, he's no longer able to drive. His son and daughter then have to take turns chauffeuring him to the supermarket twice a week while he, angry about losing his license, carps at them from the backseat about their driving.

Some of the causes are technological. Our age's innumerable medical advances—such as new drugs, improved cardiac, neurological, and vascular surgeries, breakthrough radiological techniques, and leaps in trauma and emergency care—have helped Americans achieve greater lifespans. But living longer doesn't necessarily mean living whole. Rather, technological progress enables people to postpone death but frequently leaves them with impairments that affect their abilities to walk, talk, or take care of themselves. Living longer with functional deficits means spending a larger portion of life dependent on others to help meet their basic needs. For instance, a 6-year-old boy who fell through the ice on a pond is resuscitated at a hospital emergency room and then kept alive by being placed on a ventilator for several days. Without the hospital's sophisticated machines, the child would have perished. But his brain was damaged from oxygen deprivation during his extended period in the water. Years of rehabilitation won't restore to him the prospect of being independent one day. His parents will spend the rest of their days, in the best-case scenario, having to supervise him; in the worst case, having to dress and feed and push him in his wheelchair.

Some of the causes are economic. Two decades of efforts to lower healthcare costs have worked toward shifting some of the responsibility for caring for disabled patients from professionals to families. Since acute-care hospital stays are much shorter than a generation ago, patients are discharged home generally sicker, and it's family members who are expected to take care of them. The rapid growth of home-based medical treatments—for example, home dialysis, intravenous infusions, and feeding pumps—call for greater family oversight of procedures that were previously administered only by trained hospital staff. Government programs that provide support groups, case management services, and respite care to caregivers have received better funding in the last several years but still scarcely meet the needs of the vast majority of family members with ill relatives.

A second trend that heightens the difficulties of family caregiving is that families are pulled increasingly in multiple directions. Over the past 30 years, the rise of the two-income family has meant that able-bodied American adults are on the job during working hours and therefore unavailable to be at home to take care of a sick parent, spouse, or child. (The alternative is for one of the well adults to quit working to stay home to caregive. This often means a loss of income for all family members that leaves them financially strapped.) In the past several decades, we've also been a more mobile people, less likely to live in the same town or even the same region as our closest relatives. Consequently, when a loved one becomes ill, family members who care about him the most may be scattered about the country and unable to collaborate closely on a caregiving plan.

This can distort family dynamics. Because members are so widely dispersed, the caregiving burden often falls disproportionately on the relative who lives closest to the patient. Meanwhile, it's common for the family members who live farthest away to voice the most objections to whatever caregiving plan is in place, as if to make up in power of opinion what they lack in proximity. You can be sure that, if you are the caregiver shouldering the brunt of the daily toil, this advice from afar will be not only unwelcome but also infuriating. Especially in situations in which you and your siblings from around the country must discuss a parent's care needs in tense phone conferences or testy family meetings, disagreements about who has the most right to determine the caregiving plan can cause schisms among you that may last well beyond your parent's death.

A third trend has to do with our prevailing societal ideals. Americans have always valued hard work, independence, and upward mobility. Family caregiving, on the other hand, seems nearly the antithesis of these aspirations. While it entails some of the hardest work any of us will ever undertake, it's about depending on one another, not flying solo, and digging in heels against illness's downward spiral, not climbing socioeconomic ladders. If our culture seems enamored of spending and getting, then caring for an ill loved one is about scrimping and giving. If we take pride in looking out for Number 1, then caregiving practices humility in putting number one last. All of which makes many caregivers feel out of step with American culture at large or simply "out of it"—ignored and undervalued, isolated and disconnected. You may even feel embarrassed or ashamed about what you do, convinced others may view you as practically wasting your life.

For example, the daughters of our mother with cancer will worry that some of their friends won't understand it when they're unable to make lunch dates because of their mother's frequent doctor appointments. They'll be nervous that their husbands, while abiding their attention to Mom, won't appreciate its value or applaud them for it. No one else, it will seem to them, will recognize the magnanimous efforts they make except for their mother—and even she may take the long hours they devote to her for granted.

We're increasingly likely to end up caring for an ill family member, at a time when the task has become more and more difficult for several reasons:

- Caregiving may go on for years, due to longer lifespans and advances in medical technology that leave more adults with debilitating age-related illnesses and other conditions.
- Family members are scattered geographically and have many other obligations (such as work) that compete with caregiving.
- Caregiving runs counter to the American ideals of upward mobility and independence and leaves caregivers feeling out of step and isolated in society.

All these considerations make the sacrifices of caregivers harder to sustain over time. The social systems that could serve as bulwarks for you—cohesive families or responsive healthcare professionals or even a grateful, admiring society—are often absent. It makes the toll for months or years of giving care that much steeper. And the wear and tear on you, caused by the physical and emotional burdens you bear, is already great.

To cite one old but illuminating study, published in the May/June 1989 issue of *Geriatric Nursing*, nursing professor Sandra Gaynor interviewed 87 elderly wives of neurologically impaired husbands about their caregiving experiences. Most of the wives were able to take care of their spouses, with some professional support, with relatively little hardship for the first 2 years. However, as the caregivers approached the 3-year mark, they began to report increased stress. Some had chronic back pain from lifting their husbands. Others had developed chronic sleep problems because of the many nights running that their spouses had awakened them asking for assistance getting to the bathroom or changing soiled sheets and bedclothes. (A 1998 study by the National Family Caregivers Association produced similar results, finding that 51% of the caregivers it surveyed suffered insomnia and 41% had back pain.) By year 4 in the Gaynor study, most of the wives felt unhealthy themselves and were taking prescription medications, such as anti-anxiety drugs. Few took time to safeguard their well-being in other ways.

Two important points arise from these interviews: Taking care of an ill loved one is often manageable in the short term, but the longer care is required, the more damaging is the cumulative effect. Another way of saying this is that most family members can handle a "sprint"—a short period of adrenaline-fueled, impassioned effort—but may lack the stamina to slog through a loved one's "marathon" illness. Unfortunately, many of the major medical problems that necessitate caregiving, including kidney, liver, and lung diseases, are of the grinding, uphill-and-downhill marathon variety that can sideline caregivers worn down by the course.

Fatigued runners cramp up or tucker out. Tired caregivers tend to burn out or sink. Dozens of research studies have found that family members caring for ill relatives are more prone to developing depression than their same-age peers who aren't caregiving. The studies cite that anywhere from 6 to 50% of all family caregivers are depressed, depending on whether their authors were counting mere moodiness or full-blown major depressive disorder. The latter is itself a disabling illness that usually entails intense sadness as well as the loss of the ability to enjoy favorite activities, poor sleep and appetite, and feelings of irritability, fatigue, or hopelessness. The approximately 5–10% of family caregivers who slowly descend into this state are often the ones, as Gaynor's interviews suggest, who care for a loved one for long, withering stretches. Other factors also increase your likelihood of becoming debilitated by depression: tending a patient with disruptive behavior or personality changes caused by neurological conditions; having frequent conflict with the healthcare team; and lacking available social and emotional supports. You may simply feel overwhelmed from the outset, maintaining a downcast view of the entire ordeal and of your limitations to handle it.

Whatever combination of factors leads to this state, if you end up severely depressed, you'll have less energy and creativity to bring to your labors. You may become rigid in your care routines, unable to see new possibilities for solving problems or soliciting help. Feeling trapped in an unending nightmare, you end up most vulnerable to eventually giving up. The ill loved one you care for has the greatest chance of one day landing in an extended-care facility or group home.

The second point that can be gleaned from Dr. Gaynor's interviews is that long-term caregiving is not only potentially depressing but consuming. The longer you give your all for a loved one, the less you may seem able to make time for your own needs. Life shrinks down to a narrow focus on getting through the day's feeding, toileting, and pill doling. Self-neglect breeds social isolation when you stop responding to friends' overtures. It's not unusual for caregivers to forgo medical care for themselves, even though they may be visiting doctors weekly with an ill loved one. This puts you at risk for unwittingly sacrificing your own physical health. Even if you go to your own doctor, caregiving may negatively impact your well-being. A 1999 *Journal of the American Medical Association* article reported that elderly caregiving spouses who had their own chronic illnesses were 63% more likely to die than their noncaregiving peers. A 2003 *Proceedings of the National Academy of Science* article found that family caregiving can compromise your immune system. The danger is clear: If you should break down before the relative you care for, both of you may wind up needing help from others.

The daughters aren't aware of these possible extremes. In the first days, like most family members, they feel only a vague apprehension of what's to come.

Shortly before the dinner tray arrives, a short, gray-haired social worker bustles into the hospital room. She announces that the mother's abdominal surgery to remove the mass will be scheduled in a few days and that she'll go home in the meantime. Neither the doctor this morning nor the nurses who had popped in during the day had mentioned anything about the discharge. The mother says, "All right. It will be good to get home, even for a little while." But the daughters just stare. As impatient as they are to get out of the hospital, the thought that their mother will soon be back in her small apartment makes them nervous. "Why isn't the surgery being done right away?" the older one asks. The social worker responds, "I don't know. It's the doctor's decision." When the older daughter's flustered expression remains unchanged, the social worker adds: "Cancer patients seem to do better when they're in their own homes surrounded by the people who care about them most. I'm sure she'll handle the surgery better after resting at home first."

She turns toward the mother again and says: "Your doctor will discuss the plan for the upcoming surgery and subsequent treatments with you when he gives you your discharge papers. Here's a list of home health agencies if you want to hire extra help to assist you with bathing, dressing, or maybe cleaning. I also have this patient education manual called *Coping with Cancer*." The older daughter interjects again, "What subsequent treatments are we talking about?" The social worker answers, "It's not my place to guess. The doctor will discuss it all with you." Both daughters frown. The arrangements seem haphazard and disjointed. The mother thanks her for coming. As the social worker reaches the door on her way out, she turns and asks the daughters if they have a few minutes to talk with her in the hall.

Despite the hurry she's in to meet with other patients, the social worker wants to communicate to these daughters that she understands what they're feeling. She has seen many families struggle with medical crises; she knows serious illness happens to families, not just individuals. She also knows that how family members fare is crucial to the medical outcome of the patient. It's not only that families drive patients to the appointments and badger them to follow the regimens of pills, diets, and exercises that physicians order with a flourish of pen on prescription pad. It's the intangibles that family members supply—the encouragement and humor, happy memories and favorite stories, love and a sense of purpose—that can make the difference between the ill person who sustains morale and the one who slips into pessimism. When daughters become demoralized, their mothers lose some fighting spirit. Without the patient's fighting spirit, medicine is hamstrung.

The daughters lean against the hallway railing once again. The social worker tells them empathetically she knows how hard these situations are for family members. She gives them her business card and says they can call her at any time if they have any questions about social services. She mentions the upcoming monthly meeting of the hospital's support group for the relatives of cancer patients. The daughters are just beginning to feel more relaxed with her when she adds, "If you're really worried about how your mother will do in her own residence, maybe one of you can take her into your home for a little while." They each look at her, suddenly befuddled, and say nothing for several moments. Neither of them particularly wants to have a conversation with her husband about bringing their mother home with them, though they know they should. They expect it of themselves. And they don't need to be prompted by a professional who barely knows them. The older sister finally responds in a flat voice that sounds indifferent, "We'll have to talk about it among ourselves." The social worker looks at them askance as if doubting they'll talk about it at all. Perhaps they won't follow any of her other suggestions either. She quickly wishes them luck and hurries down the hallway to meet with another patient and family.

They say nothing to their mother about the social worker's comments when they go back into the room. Mom's appetite has finally returned, and she's picking at the salad and roast potatoes on her tray. Seeing her eating gives them some reassurance that she's starting to recover from the morning's shock; it also reminds them of their promises to be home for dinner with their spouses. "We have to go. We'll be back in the morning," the older one says and bends down to hug her mother. They linger for a few minutes longer, fidgeting with the blankets, before finally shuffling out the door.

In the elevator on the way to the garage, the younger daughter says, "The social worker meant well." Her sister retorts sharply: "Everybody means well. They're full of advice and suggestions before they go running out. But she's our mother, and they expect us to make sacrifices for her." Later, as they enter the garage, the older sister says in a softer tone: "It's up to us to take care of her. Let's talk in the morning about whether we need to take her home with us. We'll take turns if we have to." The older daughter gives her sister a warm tap on the upper arm. Then the two of them climb slowly into their cars.

They drive home feeling even more greatly burdened than they did the night before. They have no intention of shirking their duties. They just want to handle them well and are not sure how.

There are tasks that the sisters will need to master to care for their mother as effectively as possible. They'll have to figure out what commitment they're willing to make to caregiving for now and then review that commitment periodically as time goes on and circumstances shift. They'll need to take advantage of all the support they can get, even if they don't think they need it and don't believe it will ease the "real" burden of taking care of their mother. They'll have to find the tenuous balance between sacrificing enough and sacrificing too much. As their mother's illness runs its course, they'll need to achieve another balance too—between hope and acceptance about what they can expect. To maintain that balance they'll need to stay aware of what's happening to everyone in the family so they can respond flexibly to changing needs. And in the midst of all of these travails, they'll have to guard against the dehumanizing loss of intimacy between themselves and the mother they love and also between themselves and their own spouses and children. Finally, they'll have to find ways to sustain the spirit by ascribing some greater meaning to this painful passage in the family's life. There's no exact order for accomplishing these tasks, but all should be thought through at some point during the caregiving ordeal. In the following chapters, we'll discuss each one, along with the challenges it poses for these daughters.

Before you can successfully undertake any of the subsequent tasks, however, you'll need to consider your level of commitment. What do you want to do? What are you realistically capable of doing? These are questions you'll probably answer differently at different times through the course of a loved one's illness. What level of commitment can you sustain for as long as the patient needs you—possibly years? Caregivers notoriously overcommit themselves and then feel trapped by promises they've made that slowly break them. Chapter 2 explores these and other questions to help you think through what you're willing and able to do so that you're comfortable with the commitments you make.

Limited Mobility Leads to Wounded Pride

Q: *My mother's arthritis has made her less and less mobile, so my family has been doing more and more of her chores and errands for her, from cleaning house to grocery shopping. This has been pretty easy to organize, and we've been able to joke her out of feeling humiliated by her dependence on us. But now her memory is really starting to go too, and she has written checks that she's forgotten to enter in her checkbook or forgotten to pay bills altogether. We know we need to start helping her with her finances, but she's very proud of having been able to take care of this since my father died. I could try to take over some of it without her being completely aware, like having some of her bills paid automatically online, but that seems so condescending I'm not sure I can pull it off. How can I broach this subject without making her feel ashamed?*

A: The fact that you're so sensitive toward your mother's feelings is in and of itself the most important factor in helping preserve her dignity as well as possible. There are other issues and strategies to consider, though, to promote this worthy goal through raising conscious awareness and choice.

A first step is clarifying her medical situation to help you better determine what aid she needs now and will in the future. The key question to pose to her physician is whether her conditions are chronic and progressive; if so, she undoubtedly will require even more of your help over time. You mentioned two separate medical problems: Osteoarthritis is generally chronic and progressive, but the degree of impairment it causes varies from one person to the next. I'd ask her physician if pain-reducing medicines and other interventions are likely to roughly preserve your mom's physical capabilities or whether she's likely to lose the ease of most of her movements. Her other condition—whose symptoms include short-term memory deficits and difficulties with concentration—is more vague. Is she suffering from early Alzheimer's dementia (chronic, progressive, and ultimately devastating), multi-infarct dementia from small strokes (whose resulting deficits may get no worse if further strokes can be prevented), or possibly major depression (whose symptoms are reversible)? Since cognitive impairment typically impacts family caregivers more than physical disability, asking her doctor to make a specific diagnosis is crucial to helping you plan ahead.

A second step may be counterintuitive: Don't shield your mother from the diagnoses and prognoses her physician makes. Trying to protect her from unwelcome news about herself that would hurt her pride would itself be infantilizing. Simply on the basis of medical ethics, your mother has the right to be fully informed about what she'll likely face. Such disclosure also has psychological utility: She'll have the information to grieve what she's losing and prepare herself for the increasing infirmity—and possible dotage—that will change her. She'll then be in a position to deliberately decide on the kind of assistance she wants now and in the future to deal with these eventualities.

Once steps one and two are completed, the third step will come much more easily: Have a discussion with her about the role she wants you and your family to play with her over time. Tell her you want to face her decline together as a family. Point out the accommodations you're already making for her and that you're prepared to do much more. Then let her guide you as to what she wants; given the circumstances, that's the best way to help her keep her dignity. If she unrealistically declines your help, saying she won't need it, gently remind her of what the doctor said. On the other hand, if she opts to go into a nursing home rather than burden you and your family, you may try to talk her out of it but should ultimately respect her right to decide how to live out the rest of her life.

How does all this translate into helping her day to day? You're already attempting to allow your mother to do as much for herself as possible. I'm sure you'll continue to strike the balance between helping her save face and helping her remain safe; you'll likely err on the side of not aiding her any more than you absolutely have to. But there still will be instances—for example, paying bills—when you'll need to confront her about her decreasing capabilities. That isn't a matter of shaming her but of gently priming her adaptation to new realities. The common medical understanding you and she will have gained may make those moments somewhat easier, but your mother will still feel mournful at those times. That's a natural response, one you shouldn't try to stop her from having. That's her best emotional means of coming to terms with the vicissitudes of age and fate.

The Guilt of the Long-Distance Caregiver

Q: *My sister has been serving as my father's part-time caregiver in a town about 2,000 miles away from me. Since I'm not there, all I can do is*

*act as an emotional support and try to provide practical advice as well. We
have different ways of coping with my father's infirmity, but we've managed
to work together on all decisions regarding his care. I have been feeling the
guilt of the long-distance caregiver while simultaneously being emotionally
drained from supporting my sister. My father seems to need more and more
care every day. My sister seems overwhelmed, and I'm frustrated that more
is not being done. Short of making repeated trips cross country, what can I do
to ensure my dad is truly getting the care he needs?*

A: The long-distance caregiver is frequently a controversial figure
in family circles. While she invariably means well, she's often maligned
by the on-site caregivers for several reasons. She's told she has no business trying to throw her weight around from afar because she's not close
enough to the situation to really understand it. When she says in her
own defense she has a job and/or family that keeps her at a distance, she's
told she should never have moved away. If she becomes so frustrated by
these criticisms that she decides to turn her back on caregiving by not
coming home or calling regularly, she's then lambasted for abandoning
her parent and siblings.

As unfair as this all seems, there are probably some germs of truth to
these criticisms. Long-distance caregivers are sometimes the offspring
who, years before, moved far away to escape their families of origin.
When aging parents become seriously ill, they do have a tendency to
charge on to the scene out of nowhere like self-styled marines hitting the
beach. If they decline providing care with the rationales they're too far
and too busy, siblings rightfully feel abandoned and angry. Yet, long-
distance caregivers have a distinct advantage that gives them an important role to play in a family's overall caregiving plan: Their distance allows them to see the forest for the trees when those closer to the scene
are too focused on the wood-grained detail of every caregiving task to
perceive how the family as a whole is managing.

It is on the basis of your more distant perspective that I'd reach out
to your sister. I'd call her or, better yet, fly home specifically to meet with
her in order to relate what you're seeing from your 2,000-mile vantage
point. After telling her how dedicated and loving a caregiving job she's
doing, broach your concerns about how father's decline is affecting your
sister's well-being. If she responds by saying you aren't there every day
and therefore don't understand, tell her that not being there every day
may actually help you more readily see the incremental changes that are
slowly occurring. If she argues that your father isn't as bad as you con-

tend, cite instances of how Dad has changed from one of your visits to the next—even if your sibling has been unaware of these changes. If your sister counters that she herself isn't struggling nearly as much as you imply, offer observations of how burnt out she sounds on the phone and appears during your infrequent visits. Above all else, tell her you love her and your father and want to do your utmost to help them, including getting your dad more help in his home or considering other living arrangements.

Keep in mind that this discussion will likely need to be repeated in subsequent conversations before your sister will trust what you're saying and embrace getting more help. Your credibility as a concerned, farsighted long-distance caregiver will depend on how well you convey that they're always close in your thoughts. Call and visit as often as feasible.

CHAPTER TWO

———————————— ∽ ————————————

Defining Commitments

When she pulls her car out of the hospital garage into the line of rush-hour traffic, the older sister takes a route past many of the important places in her family's life. There on the left is the house where she grew up and her parents lived for 40 years, one in a long row of identical two-story tar-shingled homes built after the Second World War on a once quiet avenue in a developing city neighborhood. There on the right is the tidy funeral parlor with the cramped rooms where her father's viewing took place on a rainy March night. Heading straight for another 10 minutes, she approaches the six-story red brick condominium building where her mother now lives on the second floor, the windows of her one-bedroom unit looking dark and empty among the lit blinds of the surrounding apartments. When Father died, Mother decided to sell their house because she didn't think she could take care of it by herself. Besides, she wanted to live close to her older daughter, to go shopping or drop by and have coffee with her several times a week. The apartment she purchased is so close to the daughter's own modest two-story home—around the corner, past the stop sign, down the block on the right—that Mother, when healthy, used to walk to it at a quick pace in little more than 3 minutes.

This geography traces the lives they've lived. Now the older sister wonders if there'll be new places marking unwanted changes. Will Mom still be able to walk to her home—or will the visits be one-way now, the older sister trudging to the apartment to take care of her? Or perhaps Mother will move into one of her grandkids' old bedrooms in the older sister's home. If she gets too sick to be cared for there, the city nursing home a half-mile up the road is a last resort. Where Mom ends up will be determined in part by the course of her cancer. But driving past these familiar places for the ten-thousandth time, the older sister realizes the future is partly in her hands, too. How she chooses to caregive, the commitment she makes, will have a major impact not only on where Mom spends her last days but also on the quality of the rest of her life.

These thoughts bring up a welter of feelings for the older sister, as they do for most family caregivers. She drums her fingers on the steering wheel as her mind flits from one anxiety to another: What if she commits to helping her mother but bungles it or makes decisions for her that turn out wrong? What if her strong-willed mother resents her deciding for her at all? At other times she squeezes the wheel tightly, feeling incensed about the cancer, the added responsibilities she will now have, the likelihood her mother will die anyway. She drives the car at a moderate speed, but her emotions feel like they're careening at a breathtaking pace.

You, too, may find yourself overwhelmed by strong feelings in those first days after your loved one's diagnosis. Not only are anxiety and anger common. Sadness is nearly universal. Guilt—either about not being able to do enough to help or about not really wanting to do anything at all—is also likely to torment you. The intensity of any one of these emotions would be enough to cloud your thinking at just that moment when your loved one turns to you with pleading eyes or a nurse or social worker tries to pin you down on how you're planning on helping. You'll probably find, however, you're being buffeted by several overpowering feelings at once—for example, a mixture of worry and grief or waves of anger and guilt. Being whipsawed in this way will only make thinking through your commitment to caregiving seem an impossible task.

Under this duress, many caregivers become paralyzed. Yet, in the midst of the medical crisis, your loved one and his healthcare team will be depending on you to think it through and decide. Just drifting along without making a conscious decision may eventually entrap you in others' choices and arrangements. Simply letting your emotions dictate your actions may make you balk at essential tasks at crucial moments and cause your family member to become infuriated. Somehow you need to step back and consider in a rational, deliberate fashion what you're willing to do for your loved one.

How do you contemplate your family member's illness and the prospect of caregiving in a clearheaded way? The older sister never found it easy in the past to quell her feelings, let alone make a decision about providing care. When her father became sick with cancer 10 years before, she felt so overwrought she didn't know what to do. It was a time when Alcoholics Anonymous was gaining greater public visibility and the movement's credo, "One Day at a Time," began appearing everywhere on bumper stickers. Friends explained to her that the phrase means living a life focused on handling the present to avoid being overwhelmed by concerns about the future. They convinced her she could benefit from applying this philosophy to caring for her dad. Rather than ruminating on the many nagging "what ifs" (for instance, "What if he becomes too weak to walk?" and "What if I become too tired to go on?"), she narrowed her awareness to the small details of being together and doing what needed to be done. Rather than dwelling on his medical prognosis or mounting insurance bills, she tried concentrating on doling out his next pill, scheduling his next appointment, and folding his next load of wash. By living one day at a time and reacting to each day's travails as they arose, she avoided making any overarching decisions about what she would and wouldn't do as his cancer progressed.

But now whenever she drives past the funeral parlor and remembers those awful days, she literally feels chilled. Over the course of the 7 months between her father's diagnosis and his death, she had stuck to "One Day at a Time" as his cancer filled his lungs, leaving him short of breath and exhausted, and then spread to his brain, leaving him confused. Throughout this period, focusing on the myriad daily tasks enabled her to limit her agonizing about future developments over which she had little control. Concentrating on the present also allowed her to sit and talk and take her father deeply into her heart; this still gives her some measure of solace now that he's physically departed.

However, she realizes with hindsight that living from day to day had some very negative consequences for her as well. It lulled her and made her vulnerable to later emotional turmoil. Because she'd set no clear parameters for herself for judging what she would or could do for her father and mother during his medical crisis, a kind of "mission creep" took hold as his symptoms worsened over time. At the beginning of his illness, she saw her father in his home a few days a week to take him to the doctor or help her mother with light housework. As he went downhill and his needs mushroomed, she was there every day nearly round the clock, lifting, toileting, and feeding him. Her mother was also wearing herself out. The house was a wreck because no one had the energy to clean anymore. Each day the older sister awoke with dread and each night went to bed miserable. Although physically and emotionally drained, she felt she no longer had the freedom to do anything but hang on until it was over. When her father finally died, she hated herself for feeling relieved. Afterward, it took many months for her to shake the enervating grip of more than half a year's trauma.

She recalls these events with a pained look as she steers her car around the corner of the apartment building, passes the first stop sign, and heads down the block until her own house comes into view. Seeing the yellow glow of the electric lantern at the curbside gives her a warm feeling for the first time that day that she has a home and refuge. Seeing that the kitchen lights are on brings to mind the comforting thought of the pot roast she'd set out to thaw that morning and which she hopes her husband now has simmering in the oven. She pulls the car into the driveway, turns off the engine, and then pauses for a few moments. I'll do it differently this time, she promises herself. I want to be there for Mom without losing touch with my husband and home. I'll take it a day at a time but also have a plan to guide me. Her husband opens the front door of the house and sticks his balding head out, looking at her quizzically. She hops out of the car and hurries inside.

Where the older sister turned right out of the hospital garage in the direction of the family's old home, the younger sister turns left away from it. Weaving through the evening traffic for several miles, she's soon veering onto the freeway ramp to take her to the nearby suburb where she and her husband moved into a traditional split-level 8 years ago. Once she has sped down the four-lane road across the city limit, the younger sister lowers her window as if to let the rush of suburban air clear away the fumes and frustrations of the bleak metropolis. She was affected differently than her older sister by her father's death. Her older sister became more entrenched in the old neighborhood and more involved with Mom; her life now is a virtual extension of the clannish way the family lived decades ago. But for the younger sister, her father's death spurred her to try to break with the past, to escape to a more open setting, less laden with memories. Even now she pushes hard on the gas pedal as if she can't get away from the city and her family's problems fast enough. With each additional mile she places between herself and the dismal hospital where Mom lies in the cancer ward, she feels freer and more relieved.

This is not for lack of caring. To the contrary, whenever she reflects on her father and mother, as she often does, she comes to the conclusion that she cares perhaps too much. In the history of her family, her sister was her mother's child and she was deemed her father's. Like him, she has always been quiet, pensive, and thin-skinned, lacking both the dynamism and the stalwartness her sister inherited from her mother. Also like him, she has tended to cope with stress by keeping her focus on whatever job is before her. If the older sister tried handling Dad's illness by living one day at a time, then the younger sister constricted her scope of awareness even more narrowly, proceeding with one isolated task at a time. Throughout his decline, she kept a list of things to do in her purse. Whenever Father shouted in confusion or Mother became alarmed, she resorted to pulling out the list and staring harder at the items on the paper in her hand as if this act of concentration would keep her emotions at bay. In fact, getting things done did keep her going by helping her avoid her strong feelings. But it also had the effect of making her ill prepared emotionally to deal with Dad's ultimate death. Suddenly there were no more things to do on the list—only to grieve his great loss. More than anyone else in the family, she was overcome. The older sister may have reacted with a lack of her usual energy for a few months; but she, the younger sister, had no energy or motivation for a year. At her husband's insistence, she finally went to see her family doctor. He diagnosed her with prolonged and unresolved bereavement, festering into major depression.

Racing around the tree-lined bends in the highway, the younger sister is thinking about those days and about her doctor sending her to see a female psychotherapist who was about her age. She had felt embarrassed at the time but went anyway and was surprised to find the woman helped her somewhat. The counselor mostly listened but in doing so subtly guided her to the realization that approaching the family's medical crisis one task at a time had dammed off feelings that later broke through and drowned her ability to cope. The therapist taught her that facing crises and feelings a little at a time kept the water behind the dam at a level she could withstand. The younger sister also learned that, though she'd been raised to feel responsible for those around her, she didn't necessarily need to be; her family members were capable people. This last revelation was particularly liberating. Suddenly she felt able to heed her husband's desire to move away so they could be more on their own without feeling too much guilt. She still saw her mother and sister regularly after that, but not quite as often, and the increased distance—both geographic and emotional—seemed to help her better manage her own emotions in general.

She's so deep in thought she nearly misses her exit. Cutting the wheel sharply, she deftly swings the car into the far-right lane. She glides down the exit ramp, makes a quick right onto a side street, and is plunged into a different world. High bushes shield many of the front lawns, and tall, long-limbed trees reach thickly across the roadway, making it appear in the dim light that she's traveling some dense woodland path. The sounds of the highway behind her are at once enveloped in an impenetrable quiet. As she approaches her own corner house, she allows the questions that have been hovering uneasily in the back of her mind since the night before to emerge. Will Mother's cancer drag her back to the city? Will the sense of independence she has cultivated be taken from her? Will she be thrust back into depression? She has a sudden memory of her old therapist telling her it's possible to give of yourself without losing yourself if you know how to hold your ground. This will be the main challenge, the younger sister thinks. Right now, parking the car at the curb and running across her lawn, taking her front steps two at a time, she is overjoyed to be on her own ground, far away for this night at least from the family's troubles.

Holding your ground against the press of medical events is possible only if you know your own mind, and this is harder than it sounds. Most people spend the majority of their time immersed in, rather than reflecting on, the ideas and emotions that drive their behavior. This is especially so during times of great duress, such as a family member's illness, when you're likely to be swept up in your own strong reactions. Approaching the crisis one day or task at a time, or even with a wait-and-see attitude, may help you cope temporarily by decreasing the pressure but will not provide the self-knowledge necessary to take a stand toward caregiving that's sustainable. From the outset of a family member's serious illness, you'll need to rise above your confusing feelings and contradictory thoughts by defining who you are and what committing to taking care of a loved one will mean for your life.

What exactly should you be thinking about? It's important to do a mental inventory of your thoughts and feelings about three main influences on your caregiving decision: your family and cultural backgrounds, your personal values and expectations, and your relationship with your ill loved one. In other words, you should strive to understand your outlook on family, self, and other. (We'll consider two additional influences later on.) Like the sisters, your family's history should be on your mind, especially how your relatives handled previous medical crises. But you should also reflect on how caring for one family member now and in the future may affect your ability to care for others. You'll probably also have ideas, based on religious or moral convictions, about what is the right thing to do when a loved one is seriously ill. And you'll have thoughts about how close you all are, how much you love each other, that will enter into any calculation you make about how much you should sacrifice yourself for the good of kin. One or more of these concerns—for instance, a sense of religious duty or a family tradition of caregiving—may seem to clinch your decision. But it's best to systematically mull over all three areas of influence so your ultimate choice rests on the broadest possible basis of your thinking.

How do you properly conduct such an inventory? The first step is like searching every shelf in a dark pantry to make a list of what's there. You need to look inward, scouring the cubbyholes of your mind to haul into conscious awareness hidden notions about yourself and your family, illness, and responsibility. It requires squelching self-criticism about the positive and negative attitudes you find. The second step is like planning a meal with the ingredients from that pantry. You need to assess realistically what you can accomplish with the available resources. Without meat or vegetables, you'll make no stew. Without a measure of willingness and a stock of love, you'll manage no effective caregiving.

More than anything else, doing a mental inventory requires that you set aside time for contemplation. You can undertake this by sitting in a quiet place and talking frankly with yourself about all your reactions to the prospect of providing care. You can do it more formally by writing a list of pros and cons or even composing a letter to yourself about the contents of your head and heart. If you have trouble gaining enough distance from your own thoughts and feelings to talk or write about them clearly, then unburdening yourself to a trusted friend or counselor who can act as a sounding board may help you better realize what's within you. If you understand yourself best when you contrast your ideas and emotions with those of others, then visiting caregiver support groups or online caregiver discussion groups and listening to the reactions of other family members can assist you in differentiating and clarifying your own responses. Any way you go about it, the end result should be increased insight into and acceptance of the personal strengths and limitations, idiosyncrasies, and psychological baggage you bring to the demands of ministering to a debilitated relative.

There are several ways to conduct a mental inventory of your thoughts and feelings toward caregiving, to define your commitment to it:

- Have a no-holds-barred talk with yourself about how caregiving will affect you.
- Write up a list of pros and cons.
- Write yourself a letter.
- Talk to a friend or counselor.
- Get group input, in person or online.

As they begin to unwind that evening from their trying day in the hospital, the sisters fall into their own ways of conducting inventories. Over pot roast at the kitchen table, the older sister relates in a grim tone to her husband all she heard from the doctors and nurses. He listens attentively with elbows on the table and chin propped on his hands but neither asks questions nor offers advice. Toward the end of her recitation, he nods and says in an intentionally upbeat tone, "You're strong. You sound like you're on top of things." But these words don't make his wife feel encouraged. Instead, she senses he's putting her off with a glib compliment so that he doesn't have to engage her too deeply on this topic. She thinks, This is what I get for being the person around here who does everything—a weak pat on the back but no helping hand. Then she fumes to herself, Hey, I do everything around here. Aren't I entitled to more support from him when I need it? As if he intuits what she's brooding about, her husband says sheepishly, "If you want me to go to the hospital sometime tomorrow, I'll try to get out of work for a little while." Several different reactions occur to the older sister at once: He hates going to the hospital because that's where his mother died; my mother's situation is probably bringing up bad memories for him. Isn't Mom supposed to leave the hospital tomorrow? What are we going to do with her? I'd better call my boss at the bank to see if I can get a few more days off.

"Speaking of work," her husband says, pushing back his chair, "we've got payroll due this week. I've got to go hit the paperwork." As he shuffles out of the room on his way to their basement office, his wife watches him with annoyance but says nothing.

She'd always joked to her girlfriends that she did her best thinking while washing the dishes. However much the warm, soapy water puckered her hands, it always helped her relax and focus. Fortunately, she quips ironically, her husband has left her a high stack in the sink tonight to help her concentrate her thoughts. As the running water begins producing a rising thick lather, she's already deep in reverie about what she should do. It wasn't as if she'd ever made any specific promises to her mother, she points out to herself. But she knows her mother as the pushy little woman who took care of her own mother and husband with total loyalty. She realizes her mother will expect the same kind of devoted care without question from her. At the thought of it, she scrubs each plate all the harder as if animated by the uncomfortable pressure she feels. Making sure each plate is squeaky clean before lining it up straight in the drying rack, the older sister also knows she has her own exacting standards for herself. She wants not only to do the right things but also to do them as well as they ought to be done. Shouldn't caring for your sick mother count as a right thing? she wonders. Like washing a tall mountain of encrusted dishes, it might be considered an unpleasant obligation by some, but it's necessary work that can be tolerated and even enjoyed.

After drying her hands and sitting back down at the kitchen table, the older sister thumbs through the family guide that the social worker gave her. She turns to the section on "Coping Strategies" and reads about writing down one's thoughts in different categories to help clarify priorities. On a piece of paper she rips off the "Honey Do" pad on the refrigerator, she makes three headings—"Family," "Mother," and "Me." Under the first, she quickly jots down "Loyal" and "Close." Under "Mother," she writes "Not easy," "Demanding" and "Good friend." She stares at the paper for a while before finally writing under the third heading, "Responsible—too much so." Glancing over the few words she's written, she laughs and muses to herself, With a loyal family and demanding Mom, no wonder I feel responsible for taking care of everybody. At the sound of her husband climbing the basement stairs, though, she gathers the papers up hastily. He'll just think I'm losing my nerve if he sees me doing this, she reasons. Maybe in the morning after he's gone to work and before I head back over to the hospital, I'll try writing again.

After their dinner, while waiting for the teakettle to whistle, the younger sister and her husband sit in their den talking about the day in the hospital. She says little at first other than commenting about the heat in her mother's crowded room and the way time beneath the fluorescent lights seemed to stretch into eternity. But after 30 years of marriage, her husband knows her well enough to hear the signals of greater discontent in her small complaints. She doesn't need to say much more for him to understand she's afraid of being trapped and worn down by her mother's convalescence. "You think this is pretty serious, your mother's cancer?" he asks her. "I'm not sure, but I think it is," she says hesitantly, "and I'm not sure how well I'm going to be able to handle it."

She hops up suddenly to turn off the kitchen stove and then returns with two mugs of decaffeinated Earl Grey tea. As he sips his drink, she tells him that waiting endlessly to speak with the doctors and nurses, standing in the cashier's line in the chilly hospital cafeteria, even smelling the faintly chlorinated tinge of the grayish hospital bed sheets is bringing up thoughts and feelings about her father's illness. "I can't stand the thought that Mom is going to suffer like him," she says. "I don't know if I can watch it without falling apart again." He shoots her a worried look but doesn't try to reassure her immediately. Instead he pauses before asking her to tell him more about what's scaring her. She's silent for a long while before saying, "If I get too upset about what I'm going to see, I might get depressed. If I can't take that, I'm going to have to save myself by backing away from Mom at a time when she needs me. Then I'll feel horribly guilty that I haven't come through for her." He sips his tea again before saying quietly, "You're not going to let your mother down. You're just going to do as much as you can. Your mother will understand that." She stares at her untouched cup and says, "I don't know."

They're both quiet for a few moments. He gets up to get more hot water. When he returns and sits back down on the couch, he asks, "Do you have an idea at what point you think it might be too much for you?" She says again, "I don't know." But she then adds in a low voice as if only cautiously and ashamedly putting her thoughts into words, "It'll be really bad if she needs a lot of hands-on care, like taking her to the bathroom. I also don't think I can deal with it if she goes into a coma like Dad did." He answers, "Okay, then. You can do what you can for your mother up until those points. I'll certainly help you do all you think you're able to do for her." Putting his mug down, he adds, "You probably better talk with your mother sometime about what you think you can and can't do, if it should come to those things. Talk to your sister, too." The younger sister, still speaking softly, replies, "Okay," and then takes a first gulp of her now lukewarm tea.

There are other larger influences that affect family members' commitments to caregiving. The loved one's disease itself—whether time-limited or life-threatening, slowly improving, lingering or progressing, or mildly or severely disabling—will define the very shape of the family crisis. It's the particulars of the illness that will evoke salient memories from your family and personal histories. It's the illness's passage from one phase to another that will set the demands against which you will measure your expectations of yourself. It's the duress that the illness causes that will determine whether the bonds between you and your loved one become strained. You must have some understanding of that illness to know what you may be signing on for when you consider committing to providing care.

Many family members are reluctant to know much about their relative's illness. They beg off or glaze over when healthcare professionals attempt to educate them about the disease and its treatments. Two rationales commonly are given. Some feel you're supposed to stand by your loved one regardless of how dire the medical ordeal. (Choosing to caregive only for those suffering specific conditions or only during particular phases in the course of a disease, they argue, would be like making their love conditional on biomedical circumstances.) Since they have no intention of ever backing out for any reason, it's unnecessary for them to know the details of the disease. Other family members don't want to know much because bad news heightens their anxiety to the point where they feel overwhelmed. Ignorance for them is not exactly bliss but can help them maintain their hope, even their folly.

But not having basic knowledge about the patient's illness is like driving some pitch-black country road without headlights and being jolted by every dip and thrown by every curve. Without understanding the rigors of the terrain, you're hard-pressed to prepare yourself for the ride or even judge whether you're up to the journey. It's reckless. You may not want every particular the doctors could possibly offer—indeed, knowing too much can be overwhelming. But it's essential to have at least a rough map of the illness's course so you can plan for the major landmarks and decision points on the road to recovery or demise. If solicited in small doses, the directions of healthcare professionals can be enlightening and lower, not raise, your anxiety level.

A good place to start is learning the basics about the disease from written materials that most hospitals and doctor's offices provide or from websites containing general information about the illness at hand. You'll find, once you start looking, that an overabundance of information is available. Try to stick with the most established mainstream sources—major disease-specific organizations such as the Alzheimer's Association, National Cancer Institute, and American Heart Association or reputable outlets such as familydoctor.org (run by the American Academy of Family Practice) or the American Academy of Pediatrics that provide solid, well-researched, and easily understood information. (Please see the "Resources" section for many examples.) Reading health-oriented articles in newspapers and magazines may provide you with some background but will not likely offer the breadth of understanding of a given disease that the mainstream sources do. On the other hand, reading the latest medical journals may offer highly technical information on experimental therapies that's difficult to understand and may not be pertinent to your loved one's care.

Many pamphlets and Internet resources recommend specific questions for you to pose to the patient's physician. They cover a broad range but usually include the following: What can I expect with my loved one's illness—in 1 week, a month, 3 months, a year? What are the options for treatment? What are the advantages and disadvantages of each option (such as medication side effects)? What is your reasoning for your treatment recommendations? What contingency plans do you have in mind if the initial treatments are ineffective? What role can I play in helping my sick relative? What is the best way for me to communicate with you on an ongoing basis? Should I consider getting a second medical opinion, and, if so, would you recommend another physician to me? Other, more detailed, questions will depend on the specifics of the disease and your loved one's age, history, and health. The purpose is not to become an expert in the disease and its treatments but to have some understanding of the possible options and the rationale for the physician's particular approach. You should also try to arrive at common medical objectives with the doctor—for example, saving the patient, merely slowing her decline, keeping her out of a nursing home, keeping her comfortable at home, and so on. Knowing that you and the physician are aiming for the same goal will relieve some of the pressure you'll feel and will engender greater trust in the patient's helping professionals.

Forewarned is forearmed where becoming informed about your loved one's illness is concerned—but with certain limitations. You can never really know how the illness will affect everyone until you're in the middle of it, which is why becoming aware and flexible (Chapter 6) is such an important task. Awareness will make you more nimble through the medical minefield.

Doctors vary greatly in communication styles, but many will take their cues from family members about how much information to share. If you ask the physician about the prognosis—that is, the assessment of how the patient will ultimately fare with the illness—he may resist answering you directly for fear you'll be upset with him if his prediction turns out to be wrong. But if you reassure him you want his best clinical guess and won't hold him accountable later, he'll be more forthcoming. You can also specify to doctors and nurses just how much you do and don't want to know—ranging from all available information to the gist of the matter to the barest minimum—and they'll likely accommodate your preferences. The important thing is that you glean some realistic medical picture. Forewarned is forearmed. Caregiving will be less burdensome to you over time if you are well enough informed to realize what you're getting into and can prepare yourself accordingly.

When they arrive at the hospital the next day, the sisters discover they're not prepared for what is occurring; they're less informed about their mother's illness than they'd thought. As soon as they enter her room and look at her propped up in her bed, they can see by her reddened face that she's angry. "They aren't sending me home today," she blurts out before they have a chance to greet her. She explains in a quaking voice that the surgeon came to see her very late the night before and told her that, given the ultrasound and pathology results, the cancer in her ovary had in all likelihood spread to her fallopian tubes and uterus. Rather than just having her right ovary removed, she needs to have a complete hysterectomy, he said, to extract the ovaries, the surrounding lymphatic tissue, and any other possibly malignant sites.

Instead of waiting a few days for her to regain her strength, he wants to operate posthaste. The social worker had been misinformed. Her internist had misunderstood the surgeon's note in her chart. Instead of going home today, she would soon be headed to the operating room for radical surgery.

The sisters stand there aghast. They each feel guilty that they went home and missed talking with the surgeon themselves, as if they could have protected their mother or somehow averted this treatment decision. They feel furious at the bossy social worker and the too busy internist and the general lack of communication and coordination among the healthcare team members that caused them all to be misled. Being misled only amplifies their fear that this medical crisis is out of their control. Mostly, though, they feel terrified about the surgery. Will she survive the operation? Will she be gutted and in pain? Will they get all the cancer? "Why didn't you call me last night?" the older sister asks sharply, but the mother doesn't bother responding. Both she and the younger sister know that it's just the older sister's way of giving voice to the fear they're all experiencing.

They spend most of the morning waiting for the surgeon to return so they can ask him the many questions on their minds. But he's beyond their reach in the operating room. Mother lies in her bed in an irritable mood while the sisters say little, staring blankly at the television. Nurses drift in and out every couple of hours to take Mother's vital signs, but they know nothing about the scheduling of her surgery. Angrily impatient about the lack of information by late morning, the older sister leaves an urgent phone message at the internist's office for him to call them back. At noon, just as the sisters are about to head downstairs to the cafeteria to pick up sandwiches, he startles them by striding into the room and stopping at the foot of Mother's bed, where he stands shifting his weight restlessly from one loafer to the other.

"I hear you're going to have some surgery soon," he says to the mother in a calm voice that he means to be reassuring but sounds nearly flippant. Mother forces a weak smile and replies, "That's what they keep telling me, but they don't say when or exactly what's going to happen." "I apologize for the confusion," the internist says, maintaining his calm tone. "Things change quickly here at times and then, at other times, it takes us a while to get into gear. I spoke with your surgeon late last night. He's planning a straightforward operation to take out the uterus and surrounding areas. He's done many of them. He's very qualified." He pauses briefly to look from the mother to the daughters as if to see the effects of what he presumes are his comforting words. But the mother still wears an anguished look, and the older sister is scowling. "I wish we had known that the surgery was going to be so soon and so extensive," the older sister says coldly. "What else is my mother going to have to go through? What if we want to get her a second medical opinion?"

The internist suddenly stops shifting back and forth. Sensing the older daughter's upset, he tries to speak more somberly in order to be better attuned with her mood. He explains this is all standard of care for ovarian cancer. The surgeon will cut out what he can. He will then confer with medical oncologists to make decisions about additional treatments. In most cases, the internist points out, patients undergo chemotherapy, possibly several rounds with different toxic agents; radiation therapy could also be tried if the cancer is found to have spread widely. There's no telling yet exactly what Mother will need. As for the second opinion, he explains that everyone is entitled to one—in fact, they should have one in cases of serious illness such as cancer—but the timing now is not ideal. To transfer her to another hospital to be evaluated by another surgeon, or even to see another surgeon in this hospital, would take a couple of days, and her condition demands they act quickly. "In my honest opinion," says the internist, "I think we should stick with the surgeon here. I have confidence in him." He then adds earnestly, paraphrasing his line from two nights before, "I promise we'll do everything we can. We've had some success with these combinations of treatments."

The mother and her daughters take this in silently. If things are as urgent as they sound, then a second opinion, at least about surgery, seems out. None of it surprises them, really, but hearing the doctor describe the succession of treatments brings home to them in a way they hadn't yet felt what a long, difficult fight this is going to be. The internist's use of the words "some success," while intended to be encouraging, raises in their minds the prospect of some failure. Would Mother suffer through these aggressive therapies only to die soon anyway?

The internist's pager suddenly chirps shrilly, and he gives a little jump. Twisting about quickly to turn it off, he glances at the number on the LCD screen and announces, "That's the surgeon's office calling me back. I expect they'll have some news about when your surgery is scheduled. Either I or they will call you soon with that information."

He begins moving toward the door while still facing them. "One hurdle at a time. We'll do everything we can for you," he repeats. "I'll be back to see you again soon," he calls out as he turns and exits rapidly.

As he's leaving, the older daughter looks over at her sister and then tilts her head toward the door. The younger daughter looks back at her with raised eyebrows and then begins following her sister into the hallway. "Where are you going?" their mother cries out. The older sister shouts over her shoulder, "We're going to go get those sandwiches."

At the elevator, the sisters catch up to the internist from behind. He whirls around as the older one pulls at the elbow of his white coat. "We had just one question, doctor," the older sister says. "Can you please tell us whether our mother is going to beat this cancer?" The internist, momentarily flustered by being confronted, clears his throat and says cautiously, "It's hard to say. It depends on many factors, including what the surgeon finds and the evaluation the oncologists make. We'll be in a better position to assess things down the road." The older sister reaches out and puts her hand on the physician's elbow again, this time more gently. "We're not looking for any guarantees," she tells him. "Only as much information as we can get so that we know how to plan for caring for her." He replies a little more warmly: "It all depends on how far the cancer has spread. I'm afraid ovarian cancer is often fatal because it's detected so late. For your mother to have the best chance of surviving, we have to move quickly and use all possible treatments." The older sister thanks him in a soft voice for his frankness. The elevator arrives then and he says "See you soon" as he steps on and the doors close.

If the nature of the illness affects the way family members regard their personal expectations, family backgrounds, and relationships when deciding about caregiving, then those personal and family factors also influence how loved ones view the illness. As a consequence, different family members often hear doctors' pronouncements differently and arrive at different conclusions about what caregiving might entail. This is a frequent source of conflict among family members during medical crises. You may hear the patient's prognosis as poor; others may hear it as inconclusive. They may see you as a pessimist; you may complain they're in denial. Ideally, these perspectives will be discussed among you at a time and place away from the patient and healthcare staff. Questions like "What did you hear the doctor say?" and "What's your understanding of the course of the disease?" may help you and your family members develop a common view of the medical situation. Once you're all closer in outlook about what you're facing, you're in a better position to reach agreement about how much care your ill loved one will need. Questions such as "Does Mom need help now accomplishing her daily activities?" and "Will she need more help in the future?" can help frame that aspect of the conversation. A shared understanding of those caregiving demands will allow you and your relatives to begin divvying up who should provide what essential care at what time to your sick loved one.

This raises yet another major influence on defining your commitment to caregiving—how your choice takes into account what other family members are and aren't going to do for the patient. Not all the conversations described will lead to consensus. Sometimes family members cling to divergent ideas about their loved one's medical condition, regardless of physicians' repeated explanations. Sometimes there are disputes about how much the patient should be expected to do for herself. Often the best that can be accomplished is a respectful airing of views and an empathetic agreement to disagree. In those situations one family member may decide to increase her commitment to compensate for what she perceives to be the inadequate commitment on the part of others. By the same token, some family members may back off from caregiving duties if they believe another member has committed to carrying most of the burden.

The five factors to take into account in defining your commitment to caregiving:

1. Family and cultural background
2. Personal values and expectations
3. Relationship with your ill loved one
4. The illness
5. Other family members' contributions to caregiving

After the internist's elevator departs, the sisters find they've reached such a juncture. "Forget the sandwiches," the older sister says. "I couldn't possibly eat now. Let's just go to the family lounge down the hall and talk." The younger sister nods. The lounge, filled with armchairs, old magazines, and pamphlets about diseases and hospital programs, is unoccupied. They sit down heavily on the vinyl couch at its far end. "Well, the man said it—she's going to die," the older sister announces grimly. The younger sister looks puzzled. "That's not what I heard. He said she probably will need a bunch of different treatments," the younger sister responds. "What do you think that means?" the older sister snaps back. "We've already been through this with Dad. They'll put her through one thing after another that will do little good, and then she'll die." The younger sister doesn't answer at first, but just looks at the worn carpet. She then says in a meek voice, "Well, I think we should ask him again or ask the surgeon to make sure we really know what's going to happen." The older sister just looks at her incredulously. "Well, *if* she's going to die," she says with an overly dramatic emphasis on the word "if," "I'm going to do everything I can for her until her death. I can't say I like giving up so much of my own life, but I'll do whatever it takes." The older sister looks at her sister as if waiting for her to announce her intentions.

"You know what I went through last time," the younger sister says nervously. "I'm going to have to take this a little at a time and see how well I manage. If Mom stays relatively independent, then I'll be there to support her. If she gets so sick from the cancer and all the treatments that she can't do much for herself, then I'll have to see if I'm able to continue taking care of her or whether we should look into other options."

The older sister frowns slightly. "I thought you might say something like that," she says in a low voice. "I always end up having to be the strong one. I always get most of the dirty work."

The younger sister, peeved, retorts, "You always think you have to take care of everything. You bring this on yourself. I said I'd do what I can as long as Mom is not totally dependent. You've never given me any credit."

"I have given you credit when you've actually come through," the older sister replies. "If I wasn't there for Dad at the end, he and Mom would practically have been alone."

The younger sister responds in a tear-choked voice, "That's completely untrue! I was there. You are so unfair."

The older sister looks down for a long pause as if composing herself before saying quietly, "Yes, I'm being unfair." She then stands up suddenly and says wearily, "Let's get back to the room. Mom's probably angry at us for disappearing." The younger sister slowly gets to her feet. Her older sister reaches over and squeezes her hand again and says, "We'll talk more. I'm just too worked up. I know we'll help Mom together."

Throughout their mother's illness, the two sisters would be well advised to do more than just talk again. They should periodically repeat the process of defining their commitments—doing mental inventories of their expectations, backgrounds, and relationships, learning as much as they can about Mom's medical status, and meeting together to discuss at length what's in each other's mind. As a consequence, their commitments to caregiving will be neither static promises gone stale nor obligations in which they feel entrapped. Instead, rethinking their roles and responsibilities over time will allow them to renew their vows to their loved one and rededicate themselves to the mission of providing care. It's their best means of remaining attuned to their mother's and their own shifting needs so that their evolving commitments accommodate changes in medical, psychological, and financial conditions. It's a way of striving to be realistic so that their caregiving has the greatest chance of being sustained.

Just as important as defining commitments is redefining them. You should review your commitment at regular time intervals, but also whenever changes occur that could affect the family's caregiving —a turn in the illness, a change in family circumstances or responsibilities—or you feel your own mental clarity toward or emotional reactions to your commitment shift.

Of course, even the most assiduously defined commitment to caregiving cannot be sustained without the benefit of others' support. Soliciting that support is only one part of the challenge. Feeling comfortable using the support that's available is often the more difficult endeavor. Many people balk at asking for help and feel chagrined when assistance is offered. They place their pride above pragmatism—frequently at their own peril. We'll examine these issues in depth in the next chapter.

A Tough Choice about Moving to a Nursing Home

Q: *Recently I moved my mother into a nursing home when her behavior started to scare my twin 6-year-old sons. She had lived with us for a few months and was wonderful for all of us to be around even though she needed lots of help physically. But then she started sleeping erratically. At first it was just waking a lot in the middle of the night—which was disturbing enough to the boys since she would talk to herself loudly, waking them up. I thought she was talking in her sleep, but she seemed awake, just not completely coherent. Then she began a pattern of sleeping for days, followed by staying awake for several days. During this "awake" period she would get increasingly more hostile and upset, and the boys were scared to be near her. Medication did not seem to help, and we knew this wasn't her fault, but we felt we couldn't have our whole house disrupted by this behavior. Everyone was exhausted, so we found a nice nursing home. But now I'm wracked with guilt. I feel terrible that my own children were afraid of my mother, whom I've always adored, and I feel awful that she's surrounded by strangers instead of family.*

A: Experiencing guilt in these kinds of situations is common and excruciating. None of us easily bears the feeling we've let down our loved ones, especially if we'd previously thought through and committed ourselves to providing care to them. What's a more difficult emotion for most family caregivers, though, is the deep sadness that accompanies loss. From your description, it sounds like you've suffered two significant losses. The first is the value you place on caring for all of your family members. Continuing to care for your mother in your home would have increasingly undermined your children's sense of well-being. You rightly redefined your caregiving commitment in response to greatly changed conditions; you really didn't have a choice but to take the action you did. The second is the loss of your mom herself. Dementia has transformed her. With the emotions and behaviors she displays at times, she's probably scarcely recognizable to you. She's quite possibly a stranger to herself. As emotions go, guilt tends to be a psychological cul-de-sac, leading nowhere but to further guilty ruminations. While sadness can be a harder road—rutted and slowgoing—it is a path forward. Where it leads in the best instances is to acceptance. Accepting irrevocable tragedies does have the power to assuage one's feelings of sadness and guilt. I therefore would recommend that you focus your attention on the sad feelings you surely harbor. Expressing those feelings to your children and other family members will help you all set aside memories of Mother's periods of agitation and remember instead the great loss you share. If you can bear that sadness as a family, you'll be in a better position to accept the consequences of her diseases. You can then focus on cherishing the time you had with her in your home rather than punishing yourself for not fixing what you could not prevent.

Saying "No" When Overwhelmed

Q: *For the past 15 years, I've been the primary caregiver for my wife, parents, and in-laws. My father-in-law lives 1,000 miles from us but refuses to let anyone pitch in from the outside, so every 2 months my wife stays with him while juggling her own cancer follow-up appointments. My mother, who lives nearby, is dying of complications from uncontrolled diabetes. I had taken care of both my dad and my mother-in-law before they each died. Over the past few years, my wife has had a mastectomy and undergone chemotherapy twice. Our only son recently spent a year recuperating from a major car accident, and I filled in when the home healthcare nurse couldn't take care of him. Now my father-in-law wants to live with us. When I said no, my wife called me evil and self-centered. She can't seem to see that the fear of losing her to breast cancer, along with the stress of running back and forth between two states to take care of our elderly parents, as well as our son, have totally worn me out. I have nothing left to give, and I dream of escaping it all. How do I convey this to my demanding family and make it stick?*

A: Few people reading your description of all the caregiving you've done could blame you for finally dreaming of running away— pronto. It sounds like you've given over the greater part of the past decade to loving your family selflessly and well. The irony is that it may be how steadfastly you have cared for them that has led your loved ones to regard your role as the do-everything, be-everywhere caregiver. Your long service has typecast you. It's understandable then why your wife was surprised when you declined another caregiving opportunity.

But the wording of your question suggests she was more than surprised; she seemed to be affronted. Perhaps this is because the family member to whom you finally decided to say no is her father. But I suspect there's more to the intensity of her reaction than that. If your wife were to allow herself to see that long-term multitudinous caregiving has overwhelmed you, she'd have to take into account the degree of burden her illness has placed on you. Rather than feel guilty about being a burden, she may be rigidly holding to the notions that you're not overwhelmed (only selfish) and that caregiving should be your life's fulfillment. If this is in fact her stance, it isn't a particularly empathetic one.

So what to do? You must first accept that, on your own, you aren't likely to be able to convince your wife—nor possibly anyone else in the family—you need to save yourself from endless sacrifice. It's possible others may have some sway. Your physician could write a "doctor's order" for you to cut down on caregiving to spare your health. Your minister or priest could provide a kind of moral dispensation from further caregiving in light of all the good works you've already done. But the views of these outsiders might, at best, stymie your wife's complaints but not please her. Ultimately, I believe you'll have to stand by your decision without her approval. Given how long you've been oriented to meeting others' needs, this probably will be a difficult challenge for you.

If the challenge becomes too great, remind yourself of this truism: The more you burn yourself out, the less useful to anyone you'll be. Taking steps to conserve yourself to some extent will enable you to caregive effectively, if and when you so choose. Picking your caregiving spots will work better than spreading yourself so thin that you're ripped in two.

If the logic of conserving yourself also fails to impress your wife, you can always fall back on a simple but powerful instrument: "No" means no. She doesn't have to agree with it, only respect the finality of it. Hold to it steadfastly and you'll control your own life.

Family Relations Go from Bad to Worse

Q: *I live with my 55-year-old father, who's controlling and threatens to cut me out of his will and tell my brothers and sisters that I'm doing all kinds of terrible things to him. He uses his heart condition as an excuse not to do anything for himself or to help around the house. I'm single and I refuse to use my work time to meet his needs. No other family member wants to deal with him for fear that he'll ruin their marriages. I had a relationship when he moved in, and he insisted on giving me his two cents. I need my own life back, and he needs some type of social worker. What can I do?*

A: If the best predictor of the future is the past, then our family relationships prior to a medical crisis will shape our family caregiving. Caregiver and care recipient will fight the disease together when mutual positive regard has been long-standing. But when the relationship has been characterized by mutual ambivalence, caregiving will be fraught with misgivings and mistrust, and family members will fight one another. Caregiving can provide conditions for relatives to rework previously strained relationships. (I have witnessed adult children finally win the longed-for approval of ill parents who'd always previously begrudged them such support.) But such transformations are the exception, not the rule, and you and your father are younger than many people who achieve this reconciliation. Also, when medical peril leads to increased dependence, bad relationships frequently get worse.

The tone of your question suggests your relationship with your father has been, at best, ambivalent. It probably hasn't helped matters recently that your father seems to employ whatever control he can muster over you and your siblings to extract the care he feels is owed him. He may feel justified, but you rightly feel trod upon. The guilt he incites in you will likely only hold you in thrall for so long. If you are like most family caregivers in such situations, you'll ultimately become fed up and quit.

Before that point, I'd suggest having a long, frank discussion with your father. Begin by stating that you appreciate he is your father but also acknowledge you haven't always seen eye to eye with each other. Tell him you think this may be one of those times when you may not come to agreement about what is best. Then say you want to help him during his old age but not at the expense of your own life. Ask him if he has any thoughts about how you can strike a balance between taking care of him and caring for yourself. If he reacts positively to this line of conversation, you may have some basis for caregiving in a sustainable fashion. He may agree, for instance, to hiring help to provide some of the care he needs. If he reacts negatively, though, you may have to advise him that you can no longer play the role with him he wishes.

I'd also initiate discussions with your other family members. Point out that the decision they make about providing care to your father has other ramifications—namely, affecting their relationships with you. Pushing Dad away will be tantamount to pushing you away. Coming forward to provide some help for him will amount to caring for you. Remind them that they don't have to subject themselves to their father's manipulations if they're clear in their own minds about what they're willing to offer and what liberties they aren't willing to allow him to take.

These discussions are likely to be very tough. In a best-case scenario, your father will ease up on you and your relatives will step up to help. In the worst case, Father will cry foul and your relatives will turn a deaf ear. Either way, you'll have at least taken a strong stance on what you are and aren't willing to do and what considerations you expect from your loved ones. Stating this clearly and emphatically will be your first step toward getting your own life back. Moving out of Father's house may be the second.

Afraid to Be Left Alone

Q: *My elderly aunt doesn't feel comfortable going out because her vision is very poor and so is her hearing, and now she uses a walker to get around. At the same time, she's afraid to be left alone. This causes a great deal of stress for me, her caregiver. I feel trapped. I can't even do the things I need to do, including simple errands. What can I do?*

A: Elderly people who don't hear or see well, ambulate slowly, or otherwise feel infirm in body or spirit are often difficult to coax from their homes. The irony is that some of them also don't feel safe in those havens unless someone else is present. Your aunt has become imprisoned by her fears; taking care of her has made you her hostage. What's unclear from your question are the exact workings of this trap. Is it that she insists that you—and no one else—remain home with her? Or is it that you feel compelled to be the one person who watches over her? (Perhaps both dynamics are at work.)

If the former is the case, then you can take solace in the fact she trusts and depends on you so much. Yet, in these kinds of instances, dependency can easily grow over time into overreliance on a caregiver, and a sort of obsession can take hold. It's as if the caregiver becomes a kind of talisman or good-luck charm for ensuring well-being. I've seen ill husbands have tantrums every time their well wives tried to leave the room. Those wives came to dread leaving because of the guilt they felt. It became easier for them just to stay put to avoid scenes. Of course, the more they appeased their spouses in this way, the more dependent and obsessed these husbands became with keeping them within arm's reach.

If the latter is the case, you can take pride in your commitment to your aunt. But the more you single-handedly devote yourself, the more she will expect you and you alone to take care of her. If you should happen to wear out over time and decide to recruit others to caregive to save yourself, in all likelihood your aunt will resist.

A suggestion I make to caregivers is to promote the patient's capabilities and not just her comfort. That may mean making the patient uncomfortable at times by requiring her to do more for herself or to adapt to changes in the caregiving plan. Along those lines, I'd recommend you talk with your aunt gently about how caregiving is constricting your life and then give her a choice. She can venture from the house and accompany you on your errands. Or she can accept the involvement of a home health aide on a regular basis to free up some of your time. If she balks at either choice, express your regrets to her but choose for her whichever solution works best for you. If both choices are acceptable to her, put both into operation.

In either case, you can reassure her that the changes you are making will enable you to do more of what you want—lovingly caring for her in her old age.

Balancing Financial Responsibilities with Caregiving Demands

Q: *My 75-year-old father has had a series of medical problems over the past few years, including prostate cancer, emphysema, and a near-fatal heart attack, and now has trouble caring for himself in his own home. My wife and I have offered to have him live with us, but he has other ideas. He wants one of us to cut back our work schedule to be available to him during the day and get him dressed, cook meals, and so on. We still have one child in college and are paying off a mortgage and other loans. We simply can't decrease our incomes now. But my father doesn't understand that. He thinks we're putting our material possessions ahead of family. What should we do?*

A: Money shapes caregiving, as it does most other human endeavors, by setting limits on what we can do and thereby forcing us to prioritize. Unless siblings or other family members are willing to financially support you so that you can help your dad as he chooses, you have the right to make the well-being of your immediate family your highest priority. That's not a matter of opting for materialism so much as it is fulfilling responsibilities you have to your wife and children to provide an education, reasonable shelter, and the like. Your responsibility to your father is to care for him in his old age but not necessarily on his terms.

I suggest you meet with him without your wife to have a frank heart-to-heart talk. Tell him how much you love him, but share with him the dilemma he's placing you in to choose between him and your wife and kids. Reiterate your offer to have him live with you as a way of providing for some of his needs while still allowing you to maintain your job. I suspect he will be dissatisfied with what you have to say. My hope, though, is that he'll recognize you are sincere in your efforts to compromise and that will diminish some of his anger. Even if you agree to disagree at this point, promise him you'll talk with him again in several months to see if there's been any movement from your current polarized positions that creates room for further compromise.

Other options may exist. If you call the Area Agency on Aging in your county, a counselor there can refer you to local financial planners or attorneys who specialize in the monetary issues of older people. Those professionals can discuss with you and your father such financial mechanisms as "reverse mortgages" that may allow him to remain in his home while being able to afford the hands-on support he needs. A meeting with the manager of your father's bank may also be of help. There likely are more sensible ways to meet everyone's needs other than forcing you or your wife out of work.

CHAPTER THREE

─────────── ∾ ───────────

Utilizing Support

After moving into her older daughter's house a few days after her surgery, Mother has the uncomfortable feeling she's arrived at a kind of purgatory. Her medical ordeal, she knows, is far from over; she must undergo chemotherapy as soon as her incisions heal. As weak as she already is, there's no telling when she'll be strong enough to care for herself in her own apartment. So she lies in the narrow bed in her youngest granddaughter's former upstairs bedroom, gazing in bewilderment at her strange new home. Yellowing rock posters are peeling from walls painted a fading fuchsia. Dusty stuffed animals and perfume bottles sit atop a chipped wooden bureau. She loves the spunky girl who once lived here and who's now in a distant home with a husband and baby of her own. But the fact that she's in a child's room underscores that a dramatic role reversal has occurred. She's now in a child's position, stripped by sickness of adult powers. She's no longer in charge of herself but feels instead like her daughter's burden.

The change happened so fast she didn't feel its impact until later. Two days after surgery, she was resting in her hospital bed when the social worker came in, followed by her daughters. It was obvious the three of them had been talking. The social worker announced that the mother would be leaving the hospital the next day and could go to a "sniff" (an SNF, or skilled nursing facility—that is, a nursing home) for a couple of weeks before returning to her apartment or she could go to her older daughter's house. Before the mother had a chance to answer, her older daughter had said loudly, "My mother is not going to a nursing home," and the social worker had quickly replied, "I'm glad you're willing to take her, then." When mother started to protest, the three of them had ganged up on her, and she'd relented. Perhaps if she had argued more strenuously at that point, the mother thinks now, she could have asserted her own choice. Not that she would have chosen differently, however. Even a short nursing home stay had no appeal for her. But she'd have at least felt better respected if they'd allowed her to voice her preference before pushing a decision they'd already agreed on.

Since arriving in the upstairs bedroom, Mother has felt even more like a child because of the way she's been treated by her older daughter. Her daughter has waited on her conscientiously, cooked her simple, tasty meals, and washed and folded the clothes brought over from the apartment. But she tends to fuss dramatically over every detail of her mother's care with a faintly sour expression. It's as if every bit of caregiving is an effortful task borne without joy. It's as if Mother has little other significance for her daughter these days but as a source of chores. The mother knows she's probably being too sensitive. She realizes she herself was a stern-faced fusser in her years of caring for others. It's just that being on the receiving end of her daughter's harried caretaking has quashed the little confidence the cancer hadn't already taken.

In an unguarded moment 3 days after she arrived, the mother had shared some of these feelings with her younger daughter. That child had listened intently with a concerned look but had said nothing. Now Mother finds herself worrying about what the younger daughter will do with this information. Mother would be horrified if her older daughter were to find out how she feels. Wouldn't she look like the ungrateful louse, being waited on in bed and then carping at the devoted person doing the waiting? No, she'll have to keep the feelings to herself. She rolls painfully over to her side and swears to herself that she'll pressure her younger daughter to remain quiet, too.

While Mother ruminates in discomfort, the older daughter can be heard preparing dinner downstairs. There's loud metallic clatter as she slaps a frying pan atop the stovetop burner. Then there's the rapid clop of metal on wood as she chops vegetables vigorously. To Mother's ears, it sounds like the pressured movements of an aggrieved woman. It's little wonder she fears that her older daughter is angry with her for needing care. But at that moment the older daughter is preoccupied by different concerns. It's not so much missing work and helping her mother that irks her. She just wishes she'd been told what to expect beforehand. The physical therapist at the hospital had said that Mother would be out of bed in a couple of days, and here it is 5 days later and she's still too weak to do much more than sit up. Neither therapists nor nurses warned her that her mother would also need aid getting to and from the bathroom. That has meant getting up in the middle of every night when Mother calls for her frantically to relieve herself. If the older sister had known her sleep would be so disturbed, she might have tried getting extra rest before bringing Mother home.

As she sautés onions in the frying pan with hard thrusts of the spatula, she also broods about how little support she gets for the sacrifices she's making. While her husband had acquiesced to allowing her mother to stay with them for a few weeks, he now spends his time at home holed up in the basement office, making apparent how he really feels. While her three daughters had urged her in unison to help her mom, none of them has so much as stopped by because of their busy child care schedules. And then earlier today she received a call from her sister that she found especially annoying.

After the younger sister had talked with her mom, she'd spent the next few days considering what to do. She wasn't about to confront her sister. She had no desire to either put her mother in an awkward position or make herself a target for her sister's anger. But she knew her sibling well enough to recognize the signs of trouble. Rushing around sourly, stomping about the kitchen—it could only mean that caregiving has been a strain. What made it worse was that her older sister typically played the martyr's role, insisting on taking care of everyone and then resenting when others didn't help her. If only her sister could ask directly for others' help, the younger sister thought, she wouldn't deplete herself and chafe. If only she could be convinced to approach others for support for doing her earnest best, then Mom would fare better too.

The younger sister's phone call to her older sister to discuss all this, however, went badly. When she brought up how important it is for caregiving family members to solicit others' help, the older sister had said tartly, "You mean like convince you to leave the suburbs and visit us once in a while." The very suggestion that she needed help seemed to make the older sister bristle. "We're doing fine here," she said huffily. "If others want to pitch in, I'm not going to stop them. But I'm not going to go begging them either." She added almost as a challenge, "I don't think anyone else is going to do as good a job with Mom as I am." Rather than rising to the bait, the younger sister merely sighed, promised she would try to visit more frequently, and asked her sister to please think about what she'd said. The older sister sighed then, too, before saying curtly, "Okay," and hanging up the phone.

Now as she continues preparing dinner, the older sister, frowning, replays the conversation in her mind. One part of her knows that her younger sister was only trying to help. She also knows that others' help is actually what she craves. But the greater part of her response is strongly negative, as if her sister had had the audacity to criticize her for not handling caregiving well. She is, in her opinion, a strong person, and having her mother with her for a few weeks shouldn't—and won't—get to her. Her younger sister usually bails out when things get too tough. The older sister knows she won't allow herself to bail, no matter how little support she receives.

She sticks her head out of the kitchen door and shouts up the staircase, "Dinner's in 10 minutes." The mother, musing in bed, cringes at what she hears as an angry edge in her daughter's voice. "Thank you, dear," she finally shouts back weakly after several seconds. The mother now imagines her older daughter is in a particularly bad mood. She promises herself that, when her daughter brings up her dinner tray, she'll be careful not to incite any arguments. Dealing with her daughter like this makes her stomach churn and takes away her appetite. But she tells herself she'd better eat what's on her plate or risk making her daughter angrier yet.

As a caregiving family member, you'll be forever hearing about garnering more support for the essential work you do. You'll be pressed by healthcare professionals to recruit as much help as you can in order to ward off burnout. Your friends and relatives will insist you hire someone and take time for yourself, as if cash were abundant and leisure foremost in your mind. But, as in the case of the older daughter, support, while desirable, may be problematic for you. Three types of difficulties commonly arise.

The first involves poor communication from healthcare professionals. As discussed in Chapter 2, they have a variety of styles of sharing information. Many doctors, nurses, and social workers devote themselves wholeheartedly to working with family members in the belief that doing so will positively affect their patients' recoveries and prevent their patients' relatives from developing physical or mental disorders themselves. Others pay little more than lip service to these ideas. In the rush to discharge patients from hospitals or shuttle them in and out of medical offices, they fail to take the time to educate family members adequately. Yet, others are so focused on patients' clinical conditions that they neglect to consider family members' needs at all.

These problems are borne out in a report from the United Hospital Fund of New York City entitled *Rough Crossings: Family Caregivers' Odysseys through the Health Care System*. It conducted focus groups with dozens of family caregivers to hear about their experiences with the healthcare system. Among other distressing conclusions, it found that hospital personnel communicated in a fragmented, slapdash fashion with patients' relatives. As a consequence, many of these family members became furious when, after taking their sick loved ones home from the hospital, they found they'd been poorly prepared to give pills, run intravenous pumps, use feeding tubes, and perform other caregiving tasks.

One example the report cited was of an elderly man who took his 71-year-old multiple sclerosis-stricken wife home after she'd had aggressive surgery for a life-threatening infection. None of the healthcare professionals had told him she was now incontinent. He only discovered it when he woke up in the middle of her first night back to find that she had soaked the bed. Nor had any of her providers instructed him how to change her bandages—only that it was imperative he wrap fresh dressings daily. He wound up feeling helpless. It was difficult enough caring for his wife in her disabled state without her healthcare team failing to give him the necessary information to do the job well.

If your treating professionals aren't forthcoming with information, there still may be ways you can solicit essential facts from them. Many disease-specific organizations, such as the American Heart Association and OncoLink of the University of Pennsylvania Abramson Cancer Center, have created tip sheets for educating patients and their family members about how to foster more effective communication with doctors and nurses. Other organizations have gone into the topic more exhaustively. For instance, the National Family Caregivers Association has devised an extensive training program to teach caregivers how to ask questions, take notes, and convey information about patients. The National Institute on Aging has produced a well-organized booklet entitled

Talking with Your Doctor: A Guide for Older People on how to find a doctor who will match your communication style and get the most out of your medical visit (www.niapublications.org/pubs/talking/index.asp).

Even well-informed family members, though, often feel unsupported. Information alone will provide you neither commiseration nor concrete assistance. The second problem you may encounter with support concerns the availability of emotional resources and hands-on help (such as the availability of home health aides, someone to drive to medical appointments, someone to pick up groceries, and so on). Some family members are rich in one of those resources but not the other. Both are usually needed to care for sick loved ones for extended periods of time.

What will really make you feel supported? Your fondest wish may be to have someone split the practical caregiving tasks with you. But perhaps having someone to talk to at the end of the day would lighten the load even more. Or maybe an aide with limited nursing skills has a bedside manner that makes everyone in the family feel so at ease that you're all willing and able to pitch in more on the practical necessities. Where support is concerned, the important factor in deciding what to accept is whether it's really any help to you.

In response to the caregiving you undertake, you may experience a slew of powerful emotions, including sadness, anger, and anxiety. What often makes these feelings harder to handle is when your friends and extended relatives don't grasp the seriousness of your situation or empathize with your duress. For example, the 37-year-old mother of a 16-year-old son who'd suffered a drunk driving-induced brain injury felt dismissed when other people kept telling her how "strong" she was. She didn't feel the least bit strong; she felt nearly overcome with anger and grief. She did what she did for her son, unhappily, because she felt she had no other choice. Hearing others praising her strength only convinced her they either didn't want to or couldn't hear how she was really feeling. It also conveyed to her that others thought she was strong enough to take care of her son on her own, so they wouldn't have to help. This caused her to feel isolated and much more frustrated.

Empathy is the currency of emotional support—to feel heard, understood, and cared for. If others are accurately and empathetically attuned to your feelings, you'll likely be able to better sustain yourself while shouldering heavy care burdens. If others are disinterested in your emotional reactions, you may feel deprived and depleted even if your burden is relatively light.

Most of us look primarily to our own families—spouses, parents, siblings, cousins—for empathic connection. But sometimes, because our family relationships have been conflicted or distant, our family members may not be capable of listening or understanding when we feel mired in arduous caregiving. Some of you will be resigned to this lack of emotional support; others will find it embittering. Regardless, you'll need to turn to other sources of empathy to help sustain yourself. In the best-case scenario, your loved one's or your own healthcare professionals will realize how emotionally affecting caregiving is for you, take the time to hear your reactions, and respond compassionately. Even better, attending caregiver support groups, such as those run by the Well Spouse Association, Alzheimer's Association, or local hospitals and religious groups, will give you a forum for expressing how you feel and gain the support of others in similar straits.

Finding good-hearted people to provide you with emotional support is readily possible. Finding reliable helping hands to support you logistically can be harder, at least over time. At the outset of a crisis, family members typically come together to rally around the ill loved one with promises to help one another. But as the disability drags on, some family members begin drifting back to their own personal and family responsibilities, and the care of the sick relative comes to fall on fewer and fewer members. Ultimately, in many instances, one family member does the bulk of the everyday care—feeding, soothing, lifting, dressing, cajoling, entertaining. Perhaps one or two others assist by picking up medications from the pharmacy, shopping for food, or occasionally "baby-sitting" the ill loved one so the primary caregiver can take a brief break.

Viewed as a short-term management strategy, having a small number of relatives do the hands-on work is probably the most efficient way to organize your loved one's caregiving. There's something to be said for the old expression about too many cooks spoiling the broth; the involvement of too many family members makes the numerous daily care decisions more difficult. Or, as I've heard many primary caregivers put it over the years, "No one else knows how to take care of our sick family member as well as I do since I'm the one with her all the time." But as a long-term plan, concentrating the caregiving in few hands courts disaster. If you do the vast majority of the work, you'll likely suffer the brunt of the cumulative physical and emotional toll that caregiving usually causes over months and years. If you give up the pursuits of your own life, you probably will grow gradually more resentful of the family members who still have the luxury of pursuing theirs. The danger is, without consistent logistical support, you'll burn out and then not be able to take care of your ill relative well at all.

There are two main means for you to ensure that daily practical help is available to you. The first is to take advantage of the professional care to which you're entitled. Nurse's aides and home health companions are the shock troops of our country's system of caring for its chronically and seriously ill citizens. Their purpose is to do a portion of the necessary hands-on work and thereby decrease the wear and tear of caregiving on you. They can be expensive if hired through home healthcare agencies (generally upwards of $15 per hour). When hired through newspaper ads or church recommendations, their services are usually not as costly. The second means is to delegate caregiving duties among all interested relatives. This can be achieved through periodic family meetings at which information is shared and duties divvied up. At best, these are open and honest negotiations where brothers and sisters and parents and aunts hash out who's going to do what for whom in as democratic and fair a fashion as feasible. When it works, the sacrifice is spread around, and all family members manage as well as possible through the prolonged medical crisis.

For example, a single, middle-aged father of five adult children who was steadily declining due to severe cardiac disease required daily assistance with meals and going up and down the stairs in his house. One of his children moved in with him to help him. But the other four expressed a commitment to doing all they could as well. The siblings met without Father present every several months to talk about his deteriorating condition and what caregiving tasks he needed done. They then formed a caregiving plan among themselves that included agreement about the particular tasks for which each child would take responsibility. The general plan they devised and regularly fine-tuned wasn't truly equitable. Two of the siblings had their own family problems and could only promise to pitch in minimally; the other three siblings did most of the care. But even an imperfect plan took the entire onus off the child who lived with the father and delegated responsibility just enough among them so that all of them felt supported by one another.

There are many other creative ways in which relatives can support one another. Family members can set up weekly or monthly conference calls or use a web service to set up their own chat room or a "family caregiving calendar." They can reach financial agreements that would include having each member make a monthly payment to an account to pay for support services for the patient. They can arrange for all involved relatives to have periodic and regular respites from caregiving. The possibilities are limited only by your imagination and the degree of cooperation among your family's members.

Information, empathy, and hands-on help are the kinds of support that could bolster you to handle any caregiving situation. But there's one proviso: You have to be willing to use the available supports. That brings us to the third common problem of many family members caring for loved ones. They don't take full advantage of the help they're offered. They say things like "God only gives you as much to carry as you can bear" and then tell other family members they don't need assistance. They shrug off the questions of concerned healthcare professionals about how they're coping with such glib responses as "I'm perfectly fine—it's the patient you should be worrying about." They don't allow nurses and home health companions to come to their aid, even when those services are covered by Medicare, because they say they don't like strangers coming into their homes and believe they should take care of their loved ones on their own. And yet these are the caregivers most prone to becoming careworn. Why wouldn't they use all the help they can get? The reasons for some are altruistic. They feel privileged to be in a position to make a significant difference in someone else's life and don't want to burden others with the duties involved. For others, the reasons may be more self-centered. They want to avoid experiencing the guilt they'd feel for accepting help if others were to judge them harshly for shirking their responsibilities. Even if others make no such harsh judgments, these caregivers become so identified with their heroic roles that they often condemn themselves if they display anything less than total dedication. They're also often convinced that no one else can do the job as well as they can and that other helpers just get in the way. These are people so swept up in the mission of providing care that all other considerations disappear from view. As can be seen with the older daughter, mere logic alone doesn't easily persuade them to utilize support.

If you don't like accepting help and support, why not?

Because you feel caregiving is a privilege?

Because no one else can do the job as well as you?

Because in your judgment you have more time and energy for the task than anyone else?

Because it would feel like shirking your responsibility, which would make you feel guilty?

Because you made a commitment, and making any change would feel like breaking it?

Because you've begun to define yourself solely as a caregiver?

During the following week, the older sister says nothing more to her younger sister about their tense phone conversation, but her abrupt manner indicates she's still piqued. The younger sister is perplexed about how to respond to what she perceives as the mixed message in her sister's behavior. On the one hand, her older sister becomes indignant at the slightest suggestion she needs help. On the other, she still stomps around the house carrying heaping baskets of laundry with the beleaguered look of a hard-ridden indentured servant. Perhaps the stomping is an attempt to get through to her husband, still entrenched in his basement office. Perhaps it's a plea to Mom to get stronger soon and relieve her child's burden. (With the help of physical therapy sessions in the home, Mom is getting a little stronger and can now walk slowly with a walker, although she still needs her older daughter's help with meals and getting up and down the steep stairs.) Perhaps it's the equivalent of shaking her fist at the gods for the family's medical predicament.

The younger sister is left with three bad choices: She could protect her own delicate equanimity by avoiding a confrontation with her older sister. But then she'd be pained by the ongoing spectacle of her mother wincing as her sister charges about. She could try to talk with her older sister about the emotional upheaval their mother's cancer has caused and then offer increased support. But she's afraid that will only provoke an angry, defensive reaction. Or she could try to intuit what help her sister needs. Many stoic caregivers won't ask for help because it seems tantamount to admitting defeat and losing face. Instead, it's as if they expect others to read their minds about what they need and then rush to provide it without having to be asked. But the younger sister is no clairvoyant. Without explicit direction from her sister, she's left to trial-and-error guesswork about how she should help. And if she's wrong, she's sure she'll be blasted.

The younger sister opts for the third choice anyway, hoping that her knowledge of her sister's nature will guide her safely. She stops by the house every few days with clothing and supplies she's fetched from their mother's apartment, along with groceries and toiletries she's purchased. The first time she arrives with one of these care packages, the older sister takes it grudgingly. The next time, her sister smiles faintly as if she's pleased. Feeling encouraged, the younger sister decides to take a greater chance one day. She approaches her older sister in the kitchen and offers to stay with Mom for a few hours so that her sibling can get out for errands. But the older sister stiffens at once and says coolly, "That's not necessary. I'm fine right here. No, thank you." The younger sister answers quietly, "Well, if you change your mind . . ." But the older sister has already turned away from her to face the sink full of dishes, signaling that the conversation is over.

That night, after dinner, when she and her husband take their tea in the family room, the younger sister is still aggravated by her older sister's reaction. She complains that by insisting on being in charge at all times, the older sister makes herself miserable, her husband irritated, and her mother uptight. Not that the younger sister wants to be Mom's primary caregiver, she assures her own husband. She wants to contribute, but from a safe enough distance not to become enveloped by caregiving like her sister. But she wishes they could share the labor more so everyone would feel better supported. The younger sister's husband sips once, places his mug carefully down on a coaster, and offers what is familiar advice: Write her a letter. Get your feelings out. Then decide whether or not you want to send it.

Letter writing is a common therapeutic technique that serves several purposes. For the writer, it's a means of sorting out and clarifying what you feel to better understand yourself. It's also a way to give vent to feelings that may be difficult to express or to be able to express them in a more measured form than might realistically be possible in conversation. For the reader, it's a way of learning about another's perspective and then absorbing it slowly over time. Even in an age of e-mail and instant messaging, most readers reread a written message several times before responding. It's this time delay that allows you to better take in what has been said and then to answer in a more deliberate fashion than might occur in a heated verbal exchange. In family situations in which emotions run high, such as caregiving during a medical crisis, occasional letters can help ensure that relatives listen to one another before reacting impulsively and heatedly. Communication generally becomes more civil and productive.

Before going to bed that night, the younger sister sits at her computer and taps away at the keyboard. An inveterate keeper of journals since her bout with depression 10 years before, she's accustomed to typing out whatever pops into her head to clear her mind. She writes tonight about feeling frustrated that her older sister treats her like she's incompetent. Not just now but throughout their lives—talking down to her with sometimes angry, sometimes flip, condescension. She feels herself getting angry as her fingers jump about the keys. Then she pauses, and her thoughts turn to her father. He always stood up to the older sister when he thought his youngest child was being steamrolled. She writes down a few memories of occasions when he helped her and then, as she has many times before, writes about his sickness and death. Then she thinks about his funeral and has a sudden, clear vision in her mind's eye of her older sister sobbing at his graveside. With that image, some of her anger dissipates. She remembers, as always shortly after feeling mad, that as gruff as her older sister can appear on the outside, she's just as sensitive on the inside. Still typing as thoughts occur to her, the younger sister taps out a sentence that's more concession than revelation: "My sister tries hard to do what's right even if she sometimes hurts others by the way she goes about it."

Feeling more sympathetic to her sibling now, the younger sister clicks several times on her computer screen to save tonight's free-flowing thoughts and to set up an e-mail message for her older sister. Part of the message that she writes out with care reads: "I'm not going to try to hide from you that I'm very frustrated with you now. You don't use all the help you can, and that worries me. Mom is weak now primarily because of the difficult surgery she went through. Later, if the cancer grows, she'll be much, much weaker. How are you going to manage it all then if you won't take my help or anybody else's?" She ends the e-mail on a conciliatory note: "I care about you and only want the best for all of us." Reading it back to herself, she wonders if she's been too brazen. But knowing her tendency to ruminate about things endlessly, the younger sister moves her hand quickly to click on the "Send" command, hesitates but a moment, and then whisks the message off. For whatever reaction it provokes, she figures at least she has written what she feels.

The older sister is just getting ready for bed when her husband lumbers into the bedroom and announces that she's got an e-mail message on the computer in the basement. She's surprised on several accounts—that she has received e-mail this late at night; that he has come upstairs to tell her when he wouldn't usually bother; that he has come upstairs at all, rather than continue working until she's already asleep as he's done for the past several weeks. She looks at him for clues about the message's sender or why he wants her to know about it, but he just looks back at her blandly before proceeding into their bathroom. As she puts on a bathrobe and slippers and begins heading quickly downstairs, she wonders if her husband has already read her e-mail.

Entering the basement, she scurries toward the glowing computer screen amid piles of her husband's papers on the large wooden desk. Glancing at it, she's taken aback to see a long message from her sister. Her sister rarely e-mails her. What possibly could have happened? She sits down, begins reading, and scowls. Her sister feels frustrated? Like most people wrapped up in selflessness, the older sister feels no one could be more frustrated than she is because nobody seems to understand her reasons for caring for Mom. Nor do they give her the credit she deserves, instead criticizing the hard work she does. Certainly she should accept help, she says to herself, but at a time when she decides she really needs it. It's been only a matter of weeks helping her mother; everybody's fine; it's too soon to give in.

She sits down at the desk and begins pecking out a stern reply. But, reading back what she's written after a few minutes, she doesn't like its irritable tone and cancels the message. She tries again but finds herself becoming increasingly angry. Realizing that she's too exhausted to control her emotions, she decides to respond tomorrow. After she shuts down the computer and trudges back up to her bedroom, she's surprised to find her husband in bed and awake. Did he read the message? she wonders again. "My sister e-mailed me," she announces while taking her time hanging up her bathrobe. But he simply watches her without responding. She goes on: "She wants me to get more help caring for Mom. She says I'm doing too much. She's a pain in the neck." The husband sits up in bed, clears his throat, and says in a low but firm voice: "For once, I think she's right. You've been focusing on your mother to the exclusion of everyone and everything else. I've wanted to help you, too, but the message I've gotten from you is that you have to do it all yourself." The older sister is flabbergasted. She answers in a shrill voice, "I thought you wanted to have nothing to do with my mother. That's why you're practically living in the basement." "Your mother and I have had our problems," he continues in an even tone. "But I'm worried about you. You've been running around here completely agitated like you have the weight of the world on your shoulders. It's like you think you have to save her from cancer. I've been in the basement because it's been too painful to watch. Your sister's right that you need more help." The older sister is too shocked to reply. Her husband waits for a few minutes for her to say something, but she keeps silent. He finally rolls over and faces away from her to try to sleep. She lies there fully awake for a long time, overcome with a dozen different feelings. Some are familiar: She's hurt and angry because she feels misunderstood and criticized again. Others are new: She is anxious and confused about the fact that her sister and husband seem angry with her. What are they seeing that she can't? What do they really want from her?

If you have a family member who's a do-it-all primary caregiver, there are several strategies you can use to try to help her utilize support—persuading, granting permission or dispensation, and upholding her sense of purpose. Persuasion, the means most of us naturally attempt first, is the one that's usually least effective. Because caregiving decisions are as much based on emotion as they are on reason, making a purely logical argument that getting help will sustain a caregiver (for example, "If you take care of yourself, you will have more energy to caregive") generally fails to sway her. At the same time, dramatic emotional appeals to the caregiver (for example, "You are endangering yourself by doing too much") may rock the boat but probably won't change its direction. As with the older sister, you are likely to find that exerting pressure to accept help only elicits consternation and confusion. One plea after another will be deflected. Even in those instances when you may organize enough family members to gang up on a caregiver, she may wind up cowed into making a show of using support, but your strong-arm tactics will be resented and passively resisted.

You'll probably find that a better method of encouraging a self-neglecting relative to utilize support is to grant permission or dispensation. Because many primary caregivers have a strong sense of familial obligation or moral duty that drives their need to care for their loved ones round the clock, offering them family permission (for example, "You have our blessing if you feel like you need to take time for yourself") or a kind of moral dispensation (for example, "There is no sin in caring for yourself along with your loved one") usually has greater power to influence their behavior than logical or emotionally charged arguments. There's implicit empathy in these approaches that's absent from the occasionally offensive pressure tactics of persuasion. As a consequence, most caregivers will experience your permission granting as more considerate of their values and therefore more respectful of their judgments.

It should be pointed out, though, that the impact of these approaches often depends on who's doing the granting—specifically, how much authority and emotional understanding that person has. Healthcare professionals, especially physicians, are in a unique position to counsel caregivers to accept more help by literally prescribing it as part of a wellness regimen. But as with any medical treatment, the primary caregiver has to first feel that the physician understands her before putting faith in the prescription. When physicians fail to listen first to caregivers' concerns before pressing them to utilize greater support, then caregivers will often reject their advice out of hand as inappropriate for their particular needs. An even more influential person than the physician is the ill loved one himself. When he grants permission to a caregiver, for instance, by voicing encouragement to get assistance for hands-on care, most caregivers feel a palpable reduction in guilt and obligation that would ordinarily prevent them from accepting such help. (By the same token, when a patient begs the caregiver not to leave him at any time or allow anyone else to care for him, the caregiver is going to be that much more resistant to utilizing support.)

But the most effective way for you to help a caregiving family member avail herself of support is by upholding the sense of purpose that taking care of a sick loved one gives her. Before you offer any unsolicited advice about how she should do her job, it's vital to ask her why she has chosen to do the job she's doing and what she thinks about it (for example, "Why do you devote yourself to taking care of our relative every day the way that you do? What has it been like for you?"). You need to pose these queries in a manner that doesn't suggest to the caregiver that you are calling her caregiving into question but instead conveys that you're amazed at all the things she does. When asked with genuine curiosity about their caregiving, most family caregivers will have thoughtful answers that touch on the meaning providing care has taken on in their lives (for example, "I'm doing God's work," "I'm giving back some of the love he gave me in the past," "I'm just being a good daughter"). Whatever purpose they describe, it's essential for you to honor it as a worthy mission and not challenge it as misguided. The caregiver needs to feel you're rooting for her to continue doing what she has vowed to herself to do.

If you've succeeded thus far in upholding the caregiver's sense of purpose, she'll actually give you more leeway than she otherwise might to raise questions about the methods she's employing. In particular, you can ask her if accepting greater support would further her purpose, allowing her to do more of what she's striving to do ("Do you think you can do more of God's work if you strengthen yourself with others' help?"; "Can you give more back to your loved one if you take the time to replenish yourself?"; "Can you be as good a daughter as you want to be if others support you in that effort?"). This is decidedly different from simple persuasion in which you may be trying to convince a caregiver to come over to your side of an argument about utilizing support. When you inquire about and validate the caregiver's mission first, then you're more likely to be perceived to be on her side with whatever observations or suggestions you make.

To encourage a primary caregiver to accept help, try these approaches:

- *Gentle* persuasion: Strong-arm tactics will only produce resistance, active or passive.
- Recruit an empathetic doctor: A caregiver who feels understood by the ill person's physician may be most inclined to listen to this trusted authority.
- Give permission instead of commands: Say "You have our blessing to take time for yourself" rather than "You can't keep spending every second taking care of Mom!"
- Ask instead of telling: Find out what the caregiver's sense of purpose is and then ask if utilizing help will promote that mission.
- Enlist the ill loved one: Permission to get help will have more force coming from the patient than anyone else.

On this long night, the older sister's sense of purpose has been shaken but not undermined. Her sibling's attempt at persuasion merely irritated her. Her husband's bid to confront her created more shock than change. Now as she lies sleeplessly she broods about having been wronged by them and feels less supported than ever. She'll continue to do what's important to her, she swears to herself, with or without their approval. If they really wanted to be useful, she reasons, they would help Mom and quit critiquing her. She has a mind to set both of them straight in the morning.

She hears a scraping sound from the bedroom down the hall and realizes that her mother must have gotten up and is using her walker to ambulate to the bathroom. She's surprised Mother hasn't called out for help. But then it occurs to her that her mother hasn't called out to her in the middle of the night for at least a week. Has she been going to the bathroom on her own?, she wonders with alarm. What if she fell and broke a hip? She gets out of bed and heads down the hall toward her daughter's old bedroom. Sure enough, the bedroom door is open and the bathroom door next to it is shut, with faint light visible around the doorframe. She can hear water running and the metallic clink of the walker tapping once against the formica vanity. The older sister stands awkwardly in the dark hallway for a few minutes, feeling a mixture of emotions—anxious that her mother walked on her own, embarrassed to be spying on her mother's toileting, and slightly miffed that her mother didn't seek her help. At the same time, she has an odd déjà vu feeling about checking on her daughters when they were young and needed to be tucked back into bed. When the bathroom door slowly opens and Mother pushes her walker across the threshold, her daughter says softly "Mom," and the old woman's head bobs up with a fearful look. "What are you doing here? Don't scare me like that," the mother says in a cross voice when she recognizes her daughter. "What are you doing going to the bathroom on your own?" the older sister asks. "I'm perfectly capable of going to the bathroom by myself now," the old woman replies sharply. "Why are you up? You do too much for me already. Go back to sleep."

The older sister knows that her mother, groggy and caught by surprise, is in a testy frame of mind, and her words shouldn't be taken seriously. But after the letter from her sister and lecture by her husband, her mother's retort feels like a slap in the face. She can't help reacting defensively. "What do you mean I do too much?" she demands. "You're living in my house for me to take care of you." But Mother, when riled, is more than a match for even her older daughter when it comes to bluntness. "I don't need you acting like some big shot and treating me like I'm a child," she says. "I'll be going home to my own apartment just as soon as I can."

With that, the mother pushes her walker toward the bedroom door but stops just before going inside. She turns around again and sees even in the dim light that her older daughter is upset. "I'm sorry. The pain medicine makes me tired and irritable," the mother says. "I don't mean anything by what I said." The older daughter answers quietly with a hint of hurt, "That's all right." Her mother continues, "I'm very grateful for all you've done for me. You've done everything a mother could ask for. I'm just a stubborn, independent old woman who's not used to being waited on. I get cranky, you know. That's not your fault." The mother stops to gauge the effect of her words, but her daughter just looks at her. Sensing she must make further amends, the mother continues again. "The way I can be sometimes, it's a wonder you want to take care of me at all," she says and then asks in a small voice, "Why do you do everything you do for me?" The older daughter answers without hesitation, "Because I love you. Because you've given so much to me my whole life. Because you took such good care of Dad when he was dying; you showed me what family members should do for one another."

At the mention of her husband, the mother feels a pang of sadness. "You took good care of him, too," she says. "I thank you for that, and I thank you for taking care of me now." "You're welcome," the older daughter replies. The mother pauses again, then starts inching her walker back toward the bedroom before stopping and facing her daughter once more. "I was always very proud and could never accept help from other people," she says. "That has made it more difficult for me now that I'm sick. Please do yourself a favor and let other people help you take care of me. I've got other family members, you know. Things will probably be worse for me once the chemotherapy starts, and I don't want you to have to carry all the burden." The older daughter is about to argue with her but decides it's not the time or place. She's also very tired suddenly. This conversation with her mother has relieved the tension she was feeling earlier but also has drained her emotionally. She just answers, "Okay. I'll try." The mother says "Good night" and heads into the bedroom. The older daughter waits a moment to hear her mother get settled into bed. Then she makes her way in the dark to her own bed and instantly falls asleep.

When she awakens the next day and glances at the clock, she's thrown into panic because it's already past 9:00. Her husband didn't get her up before he went to work like he always does. What about Mom's breakfast? She jumps out of bed and heads down the hallway. Her mother is already dressed and is sitting in the armchair in her bedroom, reading a mystery novel. The older daughter blurts out, "I'm sorry I overslept. Let me go get your breakfast." But Mother answers, "Bob already gave me breakfast." The older daughter, surprised, simply says "Oh." When her mother turns back to the book, the older daughter goes slowly back to her bedroom to get her robe and then goes downstairs to get coffee.

She notices she still feels very tired. Though she slept a lot last night, the weeks of tending to Mom have obviously weighed on her. She takes deep gulps of her coffee, seeking energy. But reflecting on how she's feeling this morning, she also notices that she's far more peaceful than last night. The conversation with her mother was painful in ways. It hurt to hear the comment about being a big shot, the evocation of the loss of Dad, the prediction of worse times ahead with aggressive cancer treatments. But Mom's acknowledgment of the care she's been given means a great deal to the older daughter. She feels understood and appreciated. Mom's other comment about resisting help touched her too. She knows she's like Mom; she's proud of it, in fact. So, if Mom identified that resistance as a problem she's had to overcome, then the same is likely true of the older daughter.

After placing her empty coffee cup in the sink, she goes down to the basement. She turns on the computer and rereads her sister's e-mail message. Its tone, which she had perceived last night as critical and a little haughty, today seems more caring. She's not ready to concede its main points but is willing to discuss them. She hits the "Reply" button and begins writing back to her younger sister. "I know we're both frustrated," she writes. "We should talk. How about coming over?" She then thinks for a moment and adds, "I'll ask Bob to stay with Mom tonight so we can go out. Maybe grab a bite to eat." She reads the message back to herself, shrugs, and hits "Send."

Utilizing support is crucial to sustaining you through the caregiving ordeal. But regardless of how much support you use, providing care means making sacrifices in your life and the life of your family. For some caregivers, the sacrifices become greater than they had planned when committing to providing care. As a consequence, they have trouble coping over time. Being mentally prepared to face and handle sacrifice is key to managing caregiving, especially when it may go on for years. We'll talk about that mental preparation in depth in the next chapter.

A Caregiver Needs a Doctor's Care, Too

Q: *When I accompany my mother to her neurologist's office for check-ups of her multiple sclerosis, her doctor is always quick to tell me what to do—pick up particular drugs, push my mother to avoid stress, make sure the home environment is safe for someone who is very unstable. But the doctor never asks me how I feel about doing these things or if I'm capable of managing them. How do I get the doctor to understand I have feelings and needs as well?*

A: Doctors vary greatly in the degree of attention they pay toward family caregivers. Some approach caregiving children with sensitivity, inquire about their well-being, and involve them in patients' care as trusted partners. Others seem oblivious to caregivers' concerns or order family members about as if they were deputized nurses. Physicians might be unresponsive to caregivers' needs for a variety of reasons. They may lack the training or confidence to work with "emotional" relatives or feel that doing so falls outside their medical specialty. They may feel pressed for time and therefore avoid getting into long discussions with family members for fear of prolonging the office visit. They may even be so familiar with the regimens for taking care of an ill person that they lack insight into what regular, nonprofessional people understand and can do. Without more information, it's impossible to surmise the motivations for your mother's doctor's behavior. But there are several things you can do to change your relationship with him.

There's nothing that grabs a physician's attention so much as the sight of pencil and paper. I'd suggest taking a list of your questions and observations with you each time you go to see your mother's neurologist. It will signal to the doctor clearly that you have concerns that need to be addressed before the visit's end. I've seen physicians literally snatch these lists out of caregivers' hands at the beginning of appointments, eager to quickly get through the family members' agendas. Another option is to schedule your own visit with the doctor without your mother present. You can talk frankly about your mother's prognosis, express your fears about her eventual loss of functioning, and delineate your limitations in caring for her. The doctor will understand your position better and take heed. He'll also come to know you as a person (at least to some extent). Chances are he'll never simply dictate orders to you again.

There are many other potential ways of changing you relationship with a patient's physician. On the National Family Caregivers Association website (www.thefamilycaregiver.org), you can order a pamphlet called *Improving Doctor/Caregiver Communications*. You can also learn more about the Communicating Effectively with Healthcare Professionals program that the Association has created and conducted nationally to train caregivers to get more out of their loved ones' medical visits.

Wanting to Do It All on His Own

Q: *My brother is caring for my mother, who has diabetes. No matter what I say to him, he refuses to acknowledge that he's a family caregiver. He believes the care he's providing to my mother is just part of his role as a son. I'd like to get my brother to be open to some assistance. How do I get him to realize he's a caregiver as well as a son, and, as such, can ask for help from me and others?*

A: I wouldn't put too fine a point on whether your brother defines himself as a caregiver or a caring son. Many if not most family caregivers do what they do without ever considering themselves as such. I'd suggest telling him you want to do as much as you can to enable him to succeed at his familial duties—then find a way of providing help to him so he can fulfill that mission.

I also wouldn't press him to ask for assistance. Seeking aid, for many people, feels tantamount to shirking their duties. You can argue all you like that recruiting help will allow them to caregive better, but the act of asking will still cause them to lose face. I would suggest instead that you just pitch in. Show up at your mother's house with groceries. Bring over a movie. Tell your brother you'll be there on a given day so he can go out to get his hair cut, complete errands, play a round of golf, or whatever he chooses. If he protests, politely turn his concerns aside. Don't take no for an answer. (To encourage a primary caregiver to accept help, also try the specific tips suggested on page 70.)

It'll be more challenging to convince your brother to accept professional help, such as home health aides. He will not ask for professionals on his own; you'll have to gingerly introduce them. For example, you can hire a cleaning service to come in with the understanding that he will try it for a month and then, if he doesn't like it, he can discontinue the service. In most of these kinds of cases, I've seen proud caregivers accept such services on a long-term basis once they see that the professionals involved are regular folk who really are helpful.

Of course, you'll want to be as respectful as possible of your brother's prerogatives and notions of devotion. But do take the initiative, and then sweetly cajole him for his good and your mother's.

Recognizing the Signs of Burnout

Q: *I've been providing care for 5 years to my father who suffered a moderately severe traumatic brain injury as the result of a drunk driving accident. Since last year, my sisters keep telling me that being his caregiver is burning me out and I should put him in a nursing home. They've never had a good relationship with our father because he's an alcoholic. I'm not sure whether they're giving me their advice because they're angry at him or because they're really concerned about me. I'm certainly tired, but I am not sure if I'm burning out. How would I know?*

A: "Burnout" is a popular term without a crystal-clear definition. It probably originally referred to the damage caused when an electrical appliance overheats. It was later adopted by rocketry to describe the point at which missile fuel is burned up and the missile falls back to earth. When organizational psychologists began studying the effects of chronic stress on workers, they adopted "burnout" as the word to describe the state of reduced productivity and satisfaction that those workers sometimes suffered. The missile definition may the best one to apply to long-term self-neglecting caregivers: If you spend your last stores of energy, you may then drop.

The typical signs of burnout are generally thought to include fatigue, irritability, sleeplessness, feelings of helplessness, cynicism about your job, and a tendency toward self-disparagement. It appears to overlap considerably with major depression. If you have several of these symptoms, I'd suggest making an appointment with your family doctor for a more formal evaluation. He or she may administer to you one of the many self-report measures that have been devised to assess caregivers; the best-known is the Burden Interview, created by Steven H. Zarit, PhD, and associates (available at many websites, including www.fpnotebook.com/ GER6.htm). On the basis of your score on that questionnaire, your doctor can give you feedback on how well you seem to be coping and may suggest that you need to modify your caregiving to avoid burning out.

Ultimately, though, you'll be the judge of whether taking care of your father is too much for you. It sounds as if your sisters aren't exactly objective observers. I understand their worries. If you have never attended an Al-Anon meeting for family members of alcoholics, you might find that it's an intriguing way to better understand your own motivations. Doing so would certainly please your sisters. I'd also recommend having a talk with them. Express your gratitude for their concern. Ask them to share what they've seen and heard that has been most alarming. But also raise your suspicions that their desire to protect you is linked to their wish to distance their father. If they deny it, then drop the subject. But be sure to let them know that whether or not they support your decisions is extremely important to you. With their steady encouragement, you may maintain the fire in the belly for your caregiving mission. With their constant criticism, you're more likely to go up in a puff of smoke.

Feeling Alone and Stuck

Q: *My mother suffers from renal insufficiency, which has left her needing lots of help with daily physical functioning and sometimes even mental functioning. She has to travel to the hospital for dialysis three times a week. I'm finding it very hard to find and keep supportive friends, because many people don't understand the nature of this illness or the demands of dialysis. The friends I had before my mother got sick have all disappeared. Our local congregation has not been supportive. I've looked at community support groups, but they don't seem to fit my situation. Between my full-time work, caregiving, and maintaining a household, I've been unable to keep up with the few activities I have tried. I feel stuck and am unable to think outside the box to figure out how I can reduce my isolation and find support. What can I do?*

A: There are many distressing and frustrating aspects of your caregiving situation—contending with an often little understood disabling illness and its arduous treatment; missing others' concerted caring and support; suffering exhaustion of your store of ideas. What comes across in your question, though, is the steadfastness of your commitment to caring for your mother and your continued hopes for better; otherwise you'd be shutting down in resignation rather than reaching out for new possibilities. Without knowing more about what you've already tried, it's difficult to give you advice that's germane. But I suggest you reflect on three areas of consideration.

The first involves the resources you're trying to tap. Most of us initially turn to family and local supports. If you've diligently contacted all available relatives, neighbors, church groups, and other local organizations and received insufficient responses, then, in the age of the Internet, you should try national or even international supports next. There are many websites devoted to kidney disease that could offer you and your mother medical information, chat rooms, and geographically organized contact lists. While these resources likely won't provide you with hands-on help, they can supply practical advice to replenish your store of ideas. More important, they can offer empathy from people who can understand your predicament more surely than anyone else. I've met many caregivers who've developed deep friendships with fellow caregivers in this manner, with whom they correspond on a daily basis.

The second consideration is how you've attempted to tap existing resources. While it's true that you can't squeeze blood from a stone, most of us are not surrounded by stones. We generally can derive some sustenance from the people in our lives if they're approached with the right combination of cajoling, diplomacy, and acceptance of who they are and whatever they have to offer. I'd ask yourself a series of tough questions: Am I making it as easy as I can for others to help me and my mother in the limited ways in which they're capable? Am I withdrawing my requests for help because I feel judged or pitied by them? Am I feeling rejected by them because they lack the experience to understand my situation and therefore are slow to respond? By seriously pondering the answers to these questions, you may conclude that your reactions to others' responses may have prevented you from getting any help from them at all. If this turns out to be the case, please consider trying to reach out to them again with lower expectations of their potential contributions and greater forbearance of their inadequacies.

The third consideration has to do with your mother's daily life. On the days that she doesn't go for dialysis, are there productive and satisfying roles she can still play—for instance, cooking, sewing, or even light housecleaning? If so, then it may relieve some of her dependence on you and consequently decrease the pressure you're feeling as her daughter and caregiver. The more vital her life becomes, the more revitalized you'll feel over time.

CHAPTER FOUR

———————————∽○∼———————————

Handling Sacrifice

After 2 more weeks of physical therapy, the mother announces at the kitchen table one morning she's regained enough strength to move back to her own apartment. There's no question in her voice; her firm tone says she means to go. Her older daughter looks up from her coffee, feigning surprise. She has waited for this day with a mix of feelings. Observing that her mother had barely used her walker the past week, the daughter let herself grow hopeful Mom might soon be out of her house—welcome relief from the round-the-clock responsibility for her care. At the same time, she imagined with anxiety her mother going home, tripping on her bedroom throw rug, and shattering a hip, to be found on the floor in agony hours later. As much as Mom might blame her own clumsiness in such an instance, the older daughter would still condemn herself for allowing her mother to come to harm.

With her mother watching her for a reply, the older daughter sets down her cup and makes the requisite argument. "You know you should stay with me at least until the chemo is done," she says without her usual stridency. She realizes with sadness that, if the cancer keeps growing, the treatments may never be done, stretching on round after round until Mom reaches her end. Her mother politely demurs, promising, "I'll come back here if I really need to." In her mind, she's praying that the familiarity of her own home will have a salutary effect that will help her miraculously recover—or that she'll die before she has to burden her older daughter again. Knowing her mother rarely bends, the older daughter accepts her decision as final and looks at her with admiration for grasping what may be a last opportunity to live independently on her own terms with most of her faculties and strength. As they're finishing their coffee and toast, the mother adds matter-of-factly, "Your sister has agreed to help me move back at the end of the week." The older daughter gives a start and leans forward to reply, but then thinks better of it and stops herself, getting up quickly instead to clear the dishes.

Later that morning, once the mother has gone back upstairs to rest, the older sister reaches her younger sister by phone. "You could have told me Mom was planning on going back to her apartment," she says sharply. The younger sister answers in defense, "I was honoring Mom's wishes not to tell you. I think she was afraid you'd try to stop her." She adds, trying to smooth matters over, "I know Mom appreciates the enormous amount you've done for her over the past few weeks. She just wants to lessen your burden." The older sister utters a loud, derisive "Hmm." "She'll need a lot of help to manage in her apartment," she says. "I can't be there all the time like I can in my own house. Are you planning on being there?" "I plan to do my part," the younger sister replies. The older sister answers doubtfully, "We'll see how that goes."

By the weekend, the mother is settled back into her apartment. Her daughters have neatly placed her clothes back into the drawers of the oak bureau that crowds the narrow bed in her dark bedroom. They've lined up her pill bottles along the back edge of her night table in the order in which she's supposed to take her medicines. The physical therapist had given her an aluminum cane to use when walking, but it rests against the wall in the corner of the front foyer. Instead, the mother totters slowly a few steps at a time across the thick living room carpet, leaning on couch, high-backed armchair, and cherry-wood TV console every few feet whenever she makes her way back and forth from the small kitchen. Clipped to the pocket of her white housedress is the cell phone that her daughters insist she always carry. If she falls, her children have lectured, she must use it to call them for help. If she feels suddenly ill, she must use it to call an ambulance. Having it with her also allows her daughters to call at any time to check on her and reassure themselves.

Since returning from her older daughter's home, the mother spends her days sitting in the armchair with the TV on and blinds drawn, lost in thought. Though she's lived here contentedly for 10 years since her husband died, for now the place has lost its air of coziness and comfort. She can't help dwelling on the cancer and her future; in a week, her incision will be healed enough for her to start chemo. After that, there may be a round of a different chemo. And then? Then, she says to herself, she'll feel so sick she probably won't care if she does die. As the fears cross her mind, her eyes light on the dusty framed prints on the walls—city panoramas by Sloan and profiles by Renoir that she and her husband bought—that she hasn't really looked at in ages. She notices anew the vitality of the busy street scenes, the vivaciousness of the rosy-cheeked people. Where she once identified with them, they now make her feel old and cut off from life. She stares often at the photographs of her family members arrayed on the coffee table. For the first time in years, she has begun talking out loud to the photo of her husband as a beaming, tipsy 50-year-old with a loosened tie, taken at a cousin's wedding reception, about how dearly she misses him. Eyeing the photos of her children and grandchildren, she tells herself that they have their own lives and she doesn't want to burden them. But she catches herself saying again and again, "I'd be lost without you."

The mother's move from her daughter's house to her apartment has brought other shifts. The daughters decided the older one would go back to work for now while the younger one takes a family medical leave from her job. While the older daughter still stops by daily, the new arrangement has effectively granted the younger daughter her turn to head up the caregiving. Today, when she arrives after lunch, the younger daughter drops two new women's magazines on the coffee table, bends down to press her cheek against her mother's, and then goes into the kitchen to unpack the groceries she's brought. When she returns to the living room, she's struck by the sight of her mother's slackened face and downturned mouth. If it were the older daughter who was here, she'd ignore this evidence of Mom's sadness or try to persuade her to get over it. The younger daughter, with her personal experience with depression, feels compelled to sit on the edge of the couch and pump her about how she's feeling. No, her mother says in a monotone, she's really feeling fine. No, she says, she's not sad, only very tired. The younger daughter sees that the TV is tuned to an infomercial for a men's hair replacement product and figures her mother has been totally inattentive to it. At the very least, she surmises, Mom's cancer has put her in a pessimistic fog. Slouched in her armchair, she even looks physically shrunken, her usual air of strength diminished.

The afternoon, having started off alarmingly, only becomes more trying for the younger daughter. The TV drones on, but otherwise the apartment is too quiet. She attempts to talk with her mother about old neighborhood friends, the grandchildren, even some magazine articles, but Mom gives five- or six-word answers that trail off into silence. The younger daughter makes two cups of tea, but Mom barely sips hers, idly rattling her spoon around in the saucer. The atmosphere is moribund. Her mother's mood gradually weighs on her so heavily that, by the late afternoon, she feels her own spirits flattened. When her older sister arrives around 5 o'clock, the younger daughter feels the need to share her concerns about Mom's depression. But the urge to escape from the apartment is stronger. She'll call her sister later to fill her in once she's home.

There's no escape, however, from the sense the day has gone awry. Racing down the highway at first with liberating speed, the younger daughter soon finds herself stalled in rush-hour traffic made worse by a rubbernecking delay. Arriving home after 6:30, her husband meets her at the door with a tense expression. "Had a long day with your mother?" he asks in an almost accusatory tone. She interprets this to mean "Why didn't you get home earlier to make my dinner?" She walks into the kitchen to find he's made no attempt to start dinner and has left newspapers spread out on the table. She turns to face him to complain, then decides against it and turns toward the refrigerator to pull out some hamburger meat. While the patties are broiling, she calls her sister at her house. "Mom and I had a very pleasant talk," the older sister reports nonchalantly. "I told her about the grandkids. She was telling me some things the doctors had said." The younger sister is taken aback. "Didn't she seem down to you?" she asks. "No, she was chipper," the older sister responds. "You know Mom doesn't get depressed. What are you worried about?"

The younger sister hangs up the phone mystified. She doubts her judgment could have been so off. Mother must be depressed; cancer had broken their hearts before and probably would again. Her older sister is just exceptionally oblivious. But then she begins to doubt herself. Could her sister be that unaware? Or maybe it was that Mom hadn't been depressed earlier, only quiet, and the younger daughter had misinterpreted the signs through her depressive view of the medical crisis. That was a troubling thought. She realized her tendency to see the world as gray and to expect others to view it that way too. She had to guard against her misperceptions. When she begins driving Mom to the chemotherapy suite next week, she doesn't want to mistake her mother's exhaustion for malaise. When the mother won't eat because the treatment squelches her appetite, the younger daughter doesn't want to panic that it's due to despair.

But then a more awful thought enters her mind. Perhaps Mom perked up after she left. Perhaps she just has a better rapport with her older daughter. The two of them were always closer; they may deny it, but it's true. Maybe Mom was merely tolerating the younger sister's presence and prying questions this afternoon. Mulling these possibilities, the younger sister feels a swell of anger. Why was she sacrificing her work, giving up time with her children and grandchildren, and delaying her husband's dinner if her mother doesn't value her caregiving? Why sacrifice herself if it does no one any good?

Many of us carry in our minds a kind of Platonic ideal of what a family caregiver should be—patient, generous, and strong. Some of these notions stem from popular images of respected societal figures, such as Nancy Reagan standing by her Alzheimer's-demented husband. More derive from our own experiences of how family members feel about one another and naturally tend to their own. One middle-aged woman related that years ago her mother had taken care of her ailing grandmother without complaint. Now that the mother had grown old and sick herself, she expected her daughter to take care of her in turn without complaint; the daughter held the same expectation of herself. Some ideas about what a caregiver should do and be are also rooted in religious convictions. The mother of a brain-injured teen, for example, reasoned that God had placed her daughter's disability in her path as a kind of moral test she could pass by giving her life over to caring for her child.

There are robust family members who seem to embrace these caregiving ideals. They forge ahead tirelessly over the years as if graced with exceptional stamina. Girded by resolve, they remain resilient emotionally through long periods of conflict, uncertainty, and enervating drudgery. Like efficient machines, they seem to function with focused purpose and a lack of reflection. Lifting doesn't bow them. Loss of sleep leaves them heavy-lidded but unruffled. Whether they don't feel the personal sacrifices they're making or simply don't allow themselves to attend to those feelings, they set a daunting precedent of total immersion in and dedication to providing care for their ill loved one.

But few of us can perform superhumanly for years on end with only our ideals to propel us. The reality of undertaking sacrifice is that it almost always exacts some toll. The more we choose to ignore that reality, the more that toll is compounded. The sturdiest, most gung ho caregivers may disregard the impact of dipping into their own reserves each day until that day, years later, when the cumulative depletion makes them feel sucked dry as an empty well. It's as if they're so fixed on the ideals of caring for their sick relative that they wantonly overlook that their own stock is steadily dropping. Without replenishing themselves regularly, their capacity to keep giving is reduced. They wind up losing doubly. First they choose to sacrifice many of their personal dreams and freedoms in their pursuit of caregiving. Then their abilities to caregive energetically are squandered because they've made no provisions for ameliorating the effects of sacrifice.

Family members like the younger daughter who are less idealistic about caring for a loved one frequently feel put upon by the sacrifices they are called on to make. Caregiving encumbers them like a stiff uniform; in short time, they chafe at constant duty's tight fit. As the 70-year-old husband of a woman who suffered for years with severe back pain said with black humor, "I'm incredibly good at taking care of sick people for about 48 hours. After that, they'd better recover fully or die." Giving up your time, your identity, may be grating for you as it is for most people. It's not that you don't want to do the right thing. No doubt you love your ill family member no less than the superhuman caregivers. It's that you somehow can't plunge yourself into providing care without lamenting the sacrifice of your previous life. You try to give of yourself while retaining yourself. In the best-case scenario, you manage to balance competing needs. In the worst, you are plagued with anger and guilt, sacrificing your peace of mind along with most other aspects of your life.

All caregivers—superhuman and merely human—need to be mindful of caregiving's toll and take steps to handle as well as possible the inherent sacrifices. Two means for achieving this have already been touched on. The first is conscious choice. If the younger daughter felt merely coerced into caregiving because of the urgency of the medical circumstances, her mother's high expectations of her, or her older sister's not-so-subtle demands, she would feel trapped in an imposed servitude. Every sacrifice she made on her mother's behalf would feel like a statutory sentence of hard labor. But the younger daughter found ways of making choices. Not that the medical urgency, mother's expectations, and sister's demands weren't in evidence. But within the context of those pressures, the younger sister defines her own commitment—do only what she can, short of becoming depressed. Having even that much control over a bad situation removes the sting of coercion from the sacrifices she's making. Exercising even that much volition provides her with some assurance she won't be overwhelmed and therefore helps her preserve the sense that she is yet her own person. The sacrifices are still difficult, but having consciously chosen them to an extent makes them more palatable.

The second means of handling sacrifice, discussed in Chapter 3, is garnering support. Receiving others' assistance enables you to withstand the pressures of caregiving longer. When you try to go it alone, you set yourself up for being drained slowly and continually. Like many high-energy, self-sufficient people, the older sister initially resisted allowing others to handle some of the daily caregiving chores to support her. She envisioned herself as masterfully responsible for her mother's care. Making personal sacrifices became a subconscious measure of her devotion and degree of control. Accepting help, on the other hand, seemed tantamount to declaring herself weak and losing her grip. It was only after her husband and sister confronted her that the older sister was forced to take a step back from her caregiving duties to reflect on how the sacrifices she was making were affecting her adversely. She finally conceded to spread those sacrifices around by allowing other family members to do more. In the short term, that made caregiving more bearable for her and her more bearable to everyone else. In the long term, seeking and accepting regular support will be a way for her to put water back into the well. Not surprisingly, taking in sustenance is sustaining. She'll have greater wherewithal to do more of whatever she chooses to do over time—even make more drastic self-sacrifices if her mother becomes sicker.

If choice and logistical support were everything that the younger daughter needed, she wouldn't be struggling with caregiving's sacrifices. But those elements, necessary as they are, aren't enough for her. Like many family members, she lacks certainty about what she's doing; her self-doubts add to her sense of being burdened. To buttress her ability to handle caregiving, she needs substantial emotional support as well. Emotional support can take three major forms: acknowledgment, compassion, and endorsement.

If you're the type of caregiver the younger daughter is, you need acknowledgment of your sacrifices from others. Statements such as "You're doing a lot for your mother"—so straightforward, so simple—can provide you with convincing proof that your efforts are neither invisible nor in vain. Without statements of acknowledgment, you, like the younger daughter, are likely to be left feeling ignored. You then are bound to grow bitter and disgruntled about the hard work you're undertaking. You'll be less likely to persevere over the course of your loved one's illness.

Even more than being acknowledged, caregivers like the younger daughter need to feel that others are compassionate. Awash in daily duties for years, many family members wind up feeling adrift from and forgotten by the rest of the world. Statements such as "It must be hard taking care of your mom every day" convey understanding and concern that mitigate the sense of dreadful isolation. Without feeling she's understood and cared for, the younger daughter is all the more resentful about what she has to do for her mother.

Receiving acknowledgment and compassion is essential. Receiving endorsement is ideal. Like most other caregivers, you may crave others' understanding why you've chosen to caregive; even more, you want those reasons supported. Statements such as "I can understand why you want to give something back to your mother after all she's done for you" can help you feel that your intentions, as well as efforts, are respected. When others fail to ask the younger daughter about why she gives care to her mother, she feels they're interested only in what she does, not in who she is. When they misconstrue her motives—for example, assuming she's caregiving because of guilt or for monetary gain—she feels insulted. When they grasp her reasons but argue against them—for instance, telling her she really doesn't owe her mother anything—she feels negatively judged.

It's difficult to handle any level of sacrifice if you don't receive *acknowledgment* of what you're doing for your ill loved one, *compassion* for your plight, and *endorsement* of your reasons for doing what you're doing—for who you are instead of just what you do. The fact that many caregivers don't receive all three from their family members or neighbors is why they turn to support groups and counseling.

Acknowledgment, compassion, and endorsement should be available to you to help you handle sacrifice optimally. But too often, one or more of these ingredients of psychological support are missing. Caregivers are sometimes barely acknowledged, even by other close relatives. For example, the wife of a man who was paralyzed by a stroke found that their children and her husband's siblings were so confirmed in their views that it was her responsibility solely to take care of him that they never bothered commenting on all she was doing for him.

You may also find that you're regarded with pity rather than compassion, which undoubtedly makes you feel humiliated. You'll then be much less likely to seek emotional support. For instance, the mother of a daughter with cystic fibrosis bridled at a friend's comment that her life seemed intolerable. The mother considered her life difficult, but she loved her child deeply; she felt her friend's comment reflected a complete lack of empathy for the gratification she derived from devoting herself to her daughter's care.

Sometimes caregivers are even blamed for their choices to caregive. For example, the adult sons of a mother who was caring for her second husband with severe diabetic complications said they knew she cared about their stepfather but thought she was sacrificing too much of her life for him. The mother was so keenly hurt that her sons were not supporting her caregiving decisions that she questioned whether they'd ever fully accepted her second marriage or respected her judgment.

When acknowledgment, compassion, and endorsement are not forthcoming, you should take the risk of reaching out to others to solicit those forms of emotional support. Sometimes that means attending support groups where family members commiserate about the sacrifices they make in order to bolster one another. Sometimes it means seeking out spouses or trusted siblings for heart-to-heart talks. Occasionally it means appealing to the patient herself by asking "Am I providing the help you need?" or a jocular "How'm I doing?" or even the heartfelt "Can you see how very, very hard I'm really, really trying?"

For the younger daughter, emotional support is hard to come by. She goes to bed that night convinced her mother rejects her concerns, her sister trivializes them, and her husband heeds them only after being fed. She wakes up with apprehension the next morning. She's supposed to return to her mother's apartment for what's likely to be another grueling afternoon in front of the TV. What she wants to do instead is accompany her own daughter to the mall to buy baby clothes for her sprouting 4-month-old granddaughter. That would give the younger sister joy. Sacrificing that pleasure today to endure and be endured by her mother is sheer aggravation.

After showering and dressing slowly, she picks up the phone and calls her older sister at her job. "How is Mom doing today?" she asks her. The older sister replies with irritation, "I haven't talked with her yet today. Why don't you call her? I shouldn't have to be the one to keep tabs on her." The younger sister reacts angrily. She can't stand it when her older sibling insinuates she's shirking responsibility for Mom. Her older sister never acknowledges what she does. "Did I say I expect you to be the one keeping tabs on Mom?" the younger sister shoots back. "No, no," the older sister answers in a dismissive tone. The younger sister explodes. "I'm the one who's going over there today while you're at work," she says heatedly. The older sister pauses for a long moment before saying calmly, "I don't know what's bothering you. I'm aware of what you do for Mom. This isn't some contest between us. You've caught me having a bad time at work. As a matter of fact, there's a meeting I'm already late for." The younger sister, still seething, doesn't respond. The older sister finally says, "I'll call you tonight and we can talk more about this." The younger sister replies curtly, "That'll be fine," and then hangs up.

Drifting from the kitchen to the basement and back up to her bedroom, the younger sister feels doubly miserable now. On the one hand, her sister only grudgingly gave her credit for the sacrifices she's making. On the other, she suspects she was avoiding calling Mother herself and then overreacted to what was probably just her sibling's morning mood. The younger sister morosely goes about putting away a basket of clean laundry, driving to the supermarket, and stopping at the bank, all the while keeping one eye on the clock and dreading the hour when she'll head her car downtown.

Driving hours later at a sluggish pace in the highway's far-right lane, she at first barely listens to the radio newscast because she's ruminating about how difficult the afternoon will be. Then a health segment on the broadcast mentions a cancer study, and she instantly becomes attentive. The announcer reports that their community has no higher cancer rate than the national average, despite contentions to the contrary by a local activist group. It had never occurred to the younger sister before that anybody considered her city a cancer gulch.

Several thoughts enter her mind rapidly: Perhaps breathing the local air, tainted by incinerator smoke, car exhaust, and the yeasty tinge from a beer distillery, caused Mom's cancer. Or maybe drinking the water from the lead-lined pipes in their old house caused her cells to run amok. Or maybe just the stress of crowded urban living set in motion internal processes that made her ill. Thinking of the possible causes of Mom's cancer makes the younger daughter aware that her mother must be struggling with the same kind of thoughts, contemplating how she got it, what she did wrong. That awareness is quickly followed by chagrin that she has spent so much time today in self-pity. Who is she, healthy as a horse, to complain? the younger sister berates herself. As she crosses the city line, takes the right-hand exit, and enters the slow stream of traffic, she's worked herself up to angry self-reprimands for bemoaning her inconveniences when it is Mother's life that's at risk.

She enters the apartment resolved to double her efforts to support her mom. The older woman is on the couch, wearing yesterday's housedress, as if she hasn't stirred from the spot. Her slack expression has the same look of despondency. "I went to the bank like you asked me to," the younger daughter tries cheerily. "Have you had lunch yet? Or could I make you something?" Her mother answers, "That's all right, dear. I'm not hungry."

The younger daughter, thwarted again, retreats to the kitchen to compose herself. She unloads yesterday's dishes from the dishwasher, all the while wracking her brain for ways to avoid repeating yesterday's stifled conversation. She decides to chance bringing up a topic the two have avoided for years as a way of conjuring a different time in their lives when Mother felt healthier and more capable.

Returning to the living room, the younger daughter settles next to her mother on the couch and says in a tentative voice, "Would you mind if we turned off the television?" Her mother turns to look at her quizzically, then fumbles with the remote control before the picture disappears from the screen. It occurs to the younger daughter that she feels like a young woman again about to ask her mother for advice. That's a comforting thought for her—having her mother as a guide while she plays grateful follower as if the role reversal caused by the cancer could be undone and the old order between them restored. "What was it like for you to take care of Dad when he was sick?" the younger daughter asks carefully. "How did you deal with it?"

Her mother squints as if pricked by the topic. The younger daughter is afraid she has pained her. But then her mother says in a steady monotone, "I dealt with it. What was I supposed to do? He was so sick; he needed my help. What more is there to say?" The younger daughter, caught between fear of irritating her further and eagerness to hear more, decides to press on. "Yeah, but what was it like for you?" she asks. "Wasn't it hard?"

The mother responds quickly, "You were there. You know it was hard." After pausing, she continues in a softer voice: "There wasn't anything I wouldn't do for your father. He was so sick. I was very tired by the end. I think you and your sister kept me going. I sometimes thought I couldn't keep going, but I had to."

"I don't recall you faltering," the younger daughter replies. "You seemed so strong and determined. You've always seemed so strong and determined." Her mother turns her head to look at her and answers: "I was younger then, and it was easier to be strong. Cancer scares me. I've seen what it can do. Now I'm in the position of your father. I don't like it, but I'm the one who needs the help now."

At the mention of their present predicament, the two women fall into silence for a few moments. The younger daughter is amazed that her proud mother has acknowledged needing help. But she's also wondering if Mom can hold in her mind two perspectives simultaneously— that of patient and caregiver. Can Mother really recall how draining it is to give care and empathize with the younger daughter's viewpoint? The old woman, staring ahead with a sad expression, seems momentarily unaware that her daughter is sitting next to her, let alone what she's feeling. The younger daughter brings the subject back to her father. "Did you keep going out of love? Or why?" she asks.

Mother turns to look at her again. "Of course I loved him," she answers. "But I also knew I would have to live with myself after he died; I didn't want to second-guess myself for not doing enough. That's the way I felt." Then, as if she realizes her younger daughter may be feeling similarly now, Mother adds in a low voice, "Perhaps you feel that way."

The younger daughter leans slightly toward her mom but says nothing at first. She's debating how much of her discomfort to reveal; she doesn't want to hurt her mother. But then Mom goes on. "I wish to God I hadn't put you and your sister in this position," she says. "It's lousy, I know. There's so much more you could be doing other than hanging around with a dying old lady. But I appreciate your being here anyway."

The younger daughter responds quickly, "It has been hard for me. You know how it is. But I want to be here for you. It's my choice to be here with you."

Mother makes an uncharacteristic tender gesture, reaching over and touching her daughter lightly on the wrist. "If it gets too hard, remember you can tell me," she says. "Okay," the daughter replies, unsure herself whether she ever actually would or how it would alter the caregiving she does. But she's glad for the invitation nonetheless.

Mother turns back toward the TV. "How about some lunch? Nothing too big or fancy," she says. "I brought some tuna," the daughter answers and gets up to go into the kitchen.

She feels heartened. She had thought her mom was too self-absorbed to notice her children were struggling, too. Now Mother has openly acknowledged that the younger daughter is making sacrifices. And she's attuned enough to her younger child to intuit what she's feeling. None of this changes their day-to-day circumstances. But feeling understood and appreciated has the effect of making the caregiving less oppressive for the younger sister. She makes two sandwiches quickly without feeling any resentment. On the contrary, she feels like doing more for her mother. She cuts up some fresh fruit and carefully places the slices on her mother's plate next to her tuna sandwich in a pleasing visual presentation.

When she reenters the living room with two plates in her hands, she notices her mother has flicked the TV on again and is watching with the same distant look as before. The men's hair replacement infomercial is on again. Though yesterday the daughter reacted with grave concern, this scene provokes her less now. Their conversation today reassured her that Mom hasn't entirely shut down. In fact, her mother had been present enough to make her feel understood. Now the younger daughter strives to extend to her the same degree of empathy. Who am I to insist there are better ways of coping with cancer than zoning out with TV from time to time? she asks herself. Escapism works; the younger daughter knows that firsthand. So she decides to accommodate her mom for now—with one change, however. "Do you mind if I see what else is on?" she asks as she sits down on the couch. "All right," her mother replies. Over the next hour-and-a-half, the two of them eat their tuna sandwiches and sliced fruit while enjoying an old movie starring Doris Day.

When it's time to get ready to leave, the younger daughter realizes the day was more gratifying than expected. She and her mother have always bonded with romantic comedies, but she also gleaned a clearer sense of why she is caregiving. Up until today, the big questions had gnawed at her: Why should she make these sacrifices? Will what she does matter in the end if Mother dies anyway? She had envied the ease with which her older sister finds meaning in helping Mom as her dutiful daughter. But caregiving could never simply mean saving the day or fulfilling duty to the younger sister. Her experience caring for her father convinced her she's incapable of saving anyone. And her history of becoming depressed when stressed had left her leery of upholding familial duty for duty's sake. If caregiving is to mean anything positive to her this time around, some new revelation would have to occur.

Psychological thinkers such as John Rolland, MD, and Lorraine Wright, RN, PhD, have long stressed the importance of family caregivers' beliefs. There are two dimensions to these beliefs. First, family members attribute meanings to the disease. For instance, family members may react to a loved one's diagnosis of cancer as if it's a death sentence, no matter how hopeful the doctors are. Or a family may have little concern about a loved one's diabetes, despite physicians' warnings, if other relatives have fared well with the disease and believe that this one will, too.

The second dimension has to do with the caregiving arrangements. For some, giving care to a sick relative means proving one's mettle as a true-blue family member. For others, being expected to caregive because of blood ties is an unfair burden. Between these two poles lay a host of often conflicting beliefs. You may believe that caregiving is both a sacrosanct obligation and a veritable torment. You may believe that you owe no allegiance to your relatives but feel no strain while helping out. You may be unsure about what to believe at all.

These beliefs have implications for how well you'll handle the rigors of serious illness. If you believe your loved one is going to die and your efforts will make no difference to her quality of life, caregiving's sacrifices will feel like just one more cause for suffering. But if you and your family hew to the more positive belief that your caregiving matters—contributing to a cure or at least providing solace—its hardships will be judged worthwhile and the sense of burden decreased.

Before today, the younger daughter's beliefs about the family's medical situation were largely negative. Her previous experience with cancer made her feel hopeless about her mother's prognosis. Worse, she had doubts about whether her caregiving efforts would supply either cure or solace; she was afraid they were mainly irritating. Driving home in the dim evening light, though, she reflects on what her mother said

---

Whenever you feel your sacrifices are for naught, make a list of just three things you do that make a difference—to your ill loved one, to the caregiving family as a whole, or to an individual caregiving family member. Keep in mind that these can be small differences ("Dad always finishes the homemade pie I bring, even though his aide tells me he never finishes his meals") or even the opposite of a negative ("If I didn't do . . . , Mom would . . . ").

---

and feels more positive. Not that she's any more optimistic about her mother's chances; even Mom referred to herself as "dying." But her mother's expression of appreciation has caused the daughter to reassess the value of what she's been doing. She suddenly doesn't feel so much in her sister's shadow. All her fussing and questioning did seem to give comfort. Pulling onto the highway, the younger daughter decides that her caregiving does matter. She feels clear in her mind for once that she's making some difference.

But there had been more. Rounding the bend in the road by the city line, miraculously free of heavy traffic tonight, the younger daughter replays what her mom had said about why she sacrificed so much for her husband—to avoid future guilt. The younger daughter had had fleeting thoughts in recent days along the same lines about why she had to hang in there with her mother. She knows that avoiding guilt isn't exactly a noble reason for caregiving. But she thinks to herself, if it was good enough for Mom, then it's good enough for me. Her father used to joke that guilt makes the world go round. She will try not to fail her mother during the coming days so she won't wind up condemning herself in the years ahead. Her older sister is so sure of her motivations that perhaps she doesn't need fear of guilt to help her handle caregiving's sacrifices. But balancing avoidance of guilt with avoidance of depression will have to be the younger daughter's unique way to proceed.

What attitudes about caregiving commitments and sacrifices, and the illness your loved one has, have you been exposed to in your family?

How do your own attitudes resemble or diverge from your family's attitudes?

There's no time like the present to assuage whatever guilt hasn't been avoided. As she heads down the exit ramp off the highway, she pulls over to the side of the service road and reaches into her purse for her cell phone. She knows her older sister isn't yet home from work; she'll leave her a message on her answering machine. "I want to apologize for how I snapped at you this morning," the younger sister says sincerely. "Today went much better. I feel better. Again, I'm sorry. No need to call me tonight. I'll call you from Mom's tomorrow."

In a few moments she pulls into her driveway. It's like a repeat of yesterday. Her husband greets her at the door with the same tense look. Dinner isn't in the oven, and today's newspapers haven't been removed from the kitchen table. But tonight, bolstered by a greater sense of her worth, the younger sister is in a different frame of mind. If she's going to handle caregiving's sacrifices, she says to herself, he's going to have to share in them, too. "Why don't you make your famous spaghetti and meatballs?" she says to him after heading out into the living room. "And please take the newspapers off the table while you're at it." He begins to reply but stops the instant she whirls around and gives him a look. In a few seconds, she hears him running water into the soup pot to boil. About that, at least for tonight, she feels no guilt.

Creating a strategy for handling sacrifice is essential to coping with the long-term effects of caregiving. But another question always arises: What is a realistic outcome for all the hard work you do? Many caregivers feel that realism will only make it harder to keep going. Others find that clinging to fantasies makes it more difficult to deal with a medical crisis at the end. In the next chapter, we'll weigh the psychological merits of hope and acceptance, fantasy and reality.

Carving Out an Identity Separate from Caregiving

Q: *When my mother became increasingly hunched over from osteoporosis, I wasn't sorry to move her into my home and quit my job as an interior decorator. My husband still works, and we have enough money. Besides, I stopped working for years to take care of my children when they were young; it's only right to do the same for my mom now. But I miss the creativity of decorating and the socializing with colleagues. I wish there were some way to not let my love of family completely crowd out my passion for work. Do you have any ideas?*

A: It sounds like you're looking for the means to preserve some corner of your life for interests that are entirely your own. That's a commendable goal, shared by many family caregivers, to have a source of identity and replenishment that's separate from caregiving itself. Your capacity for achieving that will depend on numerous factors, including your mother's degree of impairment, the amount of support you have from your husband and others, and your own willingness to take a hard look at the way caregiving duties currently organize your life. The key will be whether you can somehow set aside protected time for yourself that, unless some catastrophe occurs, you won't sacrifice.

There are two challenges to this—the carving out of the time and its defense. In terms of the former, I'd suggest having a talk with your mother and husband in which you inform them of your plan to work at interior decorating a few hours each week. Solicit their ideas about when it would be most convenient for them to have you unavailable to take care of their needs. However unenthusiastic they may be about your pursuit, develop a concrete plan with them about which days and hours these will be. While I don't know the interior decorating business, I'm hoping you could take on small jobs from your former employer or others that can actually be worked on just a few hours a week. That work would ideally be done outside your home so you're not within close proximity of the beck and call of your family members.

That's the easy part. The hard part is not allowing others to intrude on that time. I'm sure you'll be tested. Your mother will suddenly need you. Your husband will be hard-pressed to pitch in when he's promised. It's crucial that you hold fast. If you give up your time easily, your family will interpret that to mean resuming interior decorating isn't the high priority that you'd made it out to be and soon will be dropped. If you defend that time vigorously, particularly in the first weeks after you establish it, your family will realize you're intent on retaining some nonnegotiable aspects of your life.

Nothing is writ in stone, however. You'll have to review your plan as time goes on. Your mother may need more help at some points than at others, and you may have to trim the time you spend doing interior decorating. If your mother's condition worsens so she needs greater assistance on a permanent basis, you may have to make arrangements for her to receive aid regularly from others. But unless it stops interesting you, keep your hand in interior decorating. No one can pry your grip unless you allow it.

Teenagers: Don't Expect Too Much

Q: My dad lived by himself for years after he and my mother divorced, and he was fiercely independent, proud of doing everything for himself that Mom used to do. But then he had a mild stroke, and we had him come stay with us rather than rely on a stranger. My sisters pitch in, but they don't live that close, so it's up to me and my 19-year-old son, who's still living at home while he works and attends college part-time. My son goes out of his way to be absent whenever Dad needs help getting up the stairs to the front door or getting dressed. My father and my son don't see eye to eye on many things. My father is a former marine, and my son is, well, a typical teenager. My problem is I need my son's help emotionally and physically. My husband left me, and I need my son's brute strength to lift my father and his shoulder to lean on when I'm exhausted at the end of the day and my sisters are all tied up with their own families. How do I get him to "want" to help Dad and me?

A: When parents rue their adolescents' defiance, I often tell them that teenagers are supposed to be uncooperative; it's practically their job. It's also often the chief means by which they separate from their parents in order to forge their own identities. It's unfortunate but not surprising that your son has chosen to take his stand on the issue you care about most—caregiving your Dad. So long as this is his way of proving his independence from you and the rest of the family, I don't think you can get him to "want" to help.

You could require him to help out with some of the physical caregiving tasks, just as you might require that he mow the lawn or do other chores around the house. Like most teenagers, he'll probably resent being saddled with those responsibilities and do them, if at all, half-heartedly. Or you could try drawing on the strength of the relationship the two of you have with each other by asking him to assist with his grandfather to relieve you of some of your duress. He may not be enthusiastic about pitching in but will likely make some modest effort for your sake.

I would offer two cautions, however. It's not wise to try to play peacemaker between your father and your son. They have their own relationship with which they'll have to grapple. If anything, I would refuse to listen to their gripes about each other but instead direct them to work it out with each other. It's also not a good idea to try to use your son as a shoulder to lean on. Because he's striving in his teenage way to be more emotionally independent of you, your appeals for his support may feel especially burdensome to him and cause him to back off from you and the caregiving situation all the more.

One other thought: With his father gone and his grandfather entrenched in his home, your son may feel sad and angry about how the family has changed. That also may partly explain his resistance to helping. Counseling could assist him in coming to terms with the family changes, enabling him to handle his feelings without expressing them through negative or standoffish behaviors.

Priceless Connections—Outside the Family and In

Q: *I'm a 40-year-old wife and mother with a husband who is in a wheelchair and suffers from chronic pain as the result of a boating accident 3 years ago. He takes heavy pain medications every day. To help us out financially, my father also lives with us. He's only 62 and still works but has recently been warned by his doctor that his blood pressure is way too high and he needs to cut back to part-time. This will mean, in a sense, that I'll end up caregiving for him too, because he'll be around the house, expecting me to make him lunch and run errands for him. This can only get worse as he gets older. I have no friends and don't go out, other than to an occasional movie with my children. I'm afraid to leave the kids alone with my husband or my father, and my aunt can come over and help only once a month because of her own large family. My husband has a very bad temper and yells a lot. I feel like I'm in a cage with no way out. I'm on many medications myself, and tried counseling but had to stop because of our limited income. I live in a small town and there are no support groups around me. All I want is someone to talk to. Do you have any suggestions?*

A: The problems you mention are so various and complex that no easy advice will do them justice. But I'll offer what I can, especially something most family caregivers receive too rarely—acknowledgment. You're surely holding your family together. When your husband is not morose, your kids are not bickering, and your father is not suffering from excessive stress, I believe that in their hearts they know the debt of gratitude they owe you for the sacrifices you're making for them.

When you express that all you want "is someone to talk to," you rightly imply that connecting with others who can understand you is the best means of lessening your sense of entrapment within your family's many needs. What would be ideal for you would be contact via phone, letters, or e-mail with other caregivers of chronic pain patients. Unfortunately, the major support organizations, such as the American Chronic Pain Association, seem mostly geared for the needs of patients rather than their relatives. There are websites for faith-based organizations for chronic pain sufferers—for instance, Rest Ministries (www.restministries.org)—which do offer more family support. You may also have luck by contacting the Well Spouse Association (www.wellspouse.org) and asking to be put in touch with a chronic pain caregiver through its Mentor Program.

I'm just as concerned, though, with your connections to the people within your family. They shouldn't be like bars of a cage; they should be ties that enable you all to pull together toward a common goal—the survival and growth of all members in the face of disability. A first step in changing the quality of your family connections may be altering your expectations of others' contributions. Your father helps out financially. Do you also ask him to listen to your legitimate frustrations—or are you afraid of burdening him? Do you ask your kids to do age-appropriate house chores in order to help you—or are you concerned that having a disabled father has already deprived them?

Your relationship with your husband, of course, is the paramount connection. It isn't all right for him to yell a lot because of his pain and disability. Chronic pain patients have the same rate of depression as do long-term family caregivers—50%. Those who take opioids regularly for pain control probably have even higher rates. You mention your own medications and counseling, but it may be your husband who is depressed and needs treatment most severely. When he isn't depressed, he may have a much greater capacity to empathize with your suffering— that is, if you allow him to be your emotional partner by sharing with him the pain that you feel.

Since finances are tight, I'd suggest talking with your husband's primary-care physician about assessing him for clinical depression. A trusted pastor or priest can supply guidance for rebalancing the family relationships. Internet connections to other caregivers can provide you with free but priceless hope that things can get better.

When Senseless Tragedy Strikes

Q: *My favorite uncle, who has no kids of his own, recently suffered a severe brain injury in an accident caused by a drunk driver. His prognosis is uncertain. We don't know yet if he'll regain the abilities to see, walk, or even speak. We're all devastated, and overwhelmed by the legal bureaucracy required to ensure there are consequences that will make the driver understand the horrible impact of his actions. No one really understands what my siblings and I are living through now, and few really want to talk about it—especially because the victim is an uncle, not a parent, to us. I don't know how to cope with my pain and anger.*

A: Many of today's survivors of severe traumatic brain injuries (TBIs) from high-speed car crashes or military combat would have died years ago within hours of the calamity. Life-saving miracles for these types of patients have been produced by two decades of advances in neuroscience, trauma medicine, and neurosurgery, including intracranial pressure-relieving measures and ever more sophisticated life support systems. But miracles for the patients have often proved to be new and harrowing challenges for their close relatives. Any family member, of course, would be grateful their loved one survived brain trauma. But the odds are long that severe TBI victims will ever recover fully, despite months or years of strenuous rehabilitation efforts. In the great majority of these cases, patients are left with significant impairments in cognitive and/or physical functioning. In the most tragic instances, patients live out their years completely dependent on others, possibly in nursing home beds in near-vegetative states. It's little wonder that family members sometimes come to question medical science's benefits. For their loved one, they wonder whether he or she would have chosen to perish rather than live in so limited a fashion. For themselves, they ponder guiltily whether a loved one's earlier demise would have spared them from a heavy emotional and financial burden.

Your question put me in mind of family researcher Pauline Boss's writings on "ambiguous loss." She theorizes that, when a loved one is in a state in which he's physically present but cognitively absent (such as a coma or advanced Alzheimer's dementia), family members cannot grieve the loss because their relative is still alive. However, they cannot fully embrace him either because he is emotionally unreachable. They typically react with confusion, pain, and anger, as well as sadness, anxiety, and even terror. In that regard, what you're experiencing is normal and expectable. What is more devastating than to see someone you're so close to altered practically beyond recognition?

For this horrific situation, I'd offer two general pieces of advice. The first is to channel your anger into, rather than against, the rehab process.

Psychologist Ann Marie McLaughlin has pointed out that family members of brain injury patients are often so full of fury because of their loved ones' conditions that they need to direct their ire somewhere. More often than not, the target becomes the physicians, physical therapists, and other members of the rehab treatment team in what McLaughlin calls an "adversarial alliance." But being angry at the treatment team members will only alienate the people who are your loved one's best hopes for recovering as well as possible. Instead, make the commitment to collaborating closely with them, and turn your anger into energy for doing the hard and often repetitive work of brain injury rehab—coma stimulation exercises, muscle retraining protocols, transfers, cheerleading. Be a model of patience and determination. It will make your treatment team and loved one work harder.

It may sound paradoxical, but the second suggestion is to make your anger heard. Attending support groups made up of other victims of drunk driving will put you into contact with people who will understand the intensity of your emotions when most around you in everyday life will not. Voice your feelings; hear their concerns; share tips on coping through the worst days. The support you receive and give will make a difference. At the same time, consider writing letters to newspapers or giving community talks to communicate to the public at large about what you're going through and the critical importance of recognizing the injuries and deaths still caused by drunk drivers, even in this more enlightened age. It will help you make some meaning of what may seem a senseless injury.

When a Legacy Binds

Q: *I come from a large extended family in which most of the women are nurses and pride themselves on caring for others. I'm a nurse, too, but don't always feel like throwing myself into other people's problems. There's an elderly aunt, suffering from severe arthritis, who expects care nowadays from my three sisters and me. I have tried to avoid getting involved, but I'm getting lots of flak from my sisters and mother. They think I'm supposed to want to take care of her, especially since I'm not married. How do I deal with the family pressure and still be my own person?*

A: At some point in our lives, most of us have to deal with the tension between family legacies and individual desires. Through years of growing up, pushing limits, and eventually making compromises, we all find ways of both living our family's values in the world and pursuing our own dreams. When it comes to caregiving, however, this is a trickier balance to strike. Because the stakes are so high for a loved one with a serious or chronic illness, there's that much more pressure to take care of your own. Especially in your family, in which there's not only a powerful legacy of caregiving but also strongly held ideas about women's work, it will be more difficult to set off on a purely self-created path.

The first question I'd ask yourself is whether you believe you have the right to make decisions to direct your life. If the answer is yes, this is going to go much easier. You'll have the self-assurance to make up your own mind about whether to take care of your aunt or not. You'll be able to hear the comments from your sisters and mother for what they are—pressure tactics, heavy on the guilt, to make you choose to do what they believe you should. But you'll know that the prerogative is still yours. You can calmly turn aside their pleas if you're willing to deal with their anger. You can decide to compromise with them and pitch in a little. Or you can opt to become a full participant in whatever plans are devised to provide care to your aunt. What's most important is that you feel sure you'll make the choice. That in and of itself will give you a greater sense of control and ease your anguish.

If the answer is no—that is, you aren't confident you have the right to make your own decisions—I'd suggest stepping back and reflecting on where you are in your life. To what degree do you want your family to define you? Are you really at risk of losing the love of your relatives if you don't toe their line? These can be hard questions to think through. A good friend—someone outside of the family—may be able to help you clarify your thoughts and feelings. Psychotherapists specialize in working as partners on this kind of endeavor—helping you be all that you want to be.

Going It Alone

Q: *After my husband died 5 years ago, my older brother moved into my house. He never got married, and I never had children. Now we are the only remaining members of our small immediate family. In the past 2 years, my brother has been very forgetful and showing signs of dementia. I've done all I can to help him, including staying up with him in the middle of every night trying to calm him down. I'm so exhausted now that I can barely function. The problem is that I have no other family members to help me with the caregiving. What can I do to handle all this without any family to support me?*

A: Your brother is very fortunate to have you. You're making sacrifices that might be expected of a spouse or a child but that most siblings don't even attempt. The sacrifices are undoubtedly harder without another family member to at least cheer you on. There may be medical, social service, and community interventions that, though a poor substitute for family, may make your job easier.

Medically, your brother is displaying short-term memory problems, periods of agitation, and reversal of his sleep–wake cycle. These symptoms are consistent with a diagnosis of Alzheimer's dementia, Stage II. While we don't yet have the remedies to halt the progression of this terrible disease, we do have medications, such as antidepressants, antipsychotics, and cholinesterase inhibitors, to mitigate your brother's behavioral problems and improve his sleep so you can get some rest. If you haven't already done so, it would be essential to have your brother evaluated by a family physician, neurologist, or geriatric psychiatrist. As his dementia progresses, it's likely he'll move into Stage III, during which he'll be much more docile. But he'll also be far less independent at that point and in all likelihood will eventually need to be placed in a nursing home.

The social services available to you will depend on what's offered in your county, either through your Area Agency on Aging or a branch of the Alzheimer's Association. Ideally, there should be a day program for your brother several times a week, home health aides, a Meals on Wheels program, and a caregiver support program to offer you counseling and case management. Friends, neighbors, and church members are also often of great assistance for providing brief respites and hands-on help with home upkeep.

Neither professionals nor community members will give you the love and loyalty typically provided by family. I'm sure that makes you feel alone at times. But there's a modicum of caring and devotion available for most caregivers. If you cobble together medical, social service, and community resources into the safety net of a quasi family, then you'll feel better supported.

At the Breaking Point

Q: *Sometimes when I am very tired or frustrated, I lose patience and am rough with my mother. I know it isn't her fault that she's disabled, but, nevertheless, her disability manifests itself in her body, so that is where I focus my emotions. I want to shake her, and sometimes I do. I scare myself sometimes, and then I feel guilty and want to cry. I do understand how a family*

*caregiver can be moved to what might seem like abusive action by someone
else. How do I handle my emotions when I feel as if they are about to get the
better of me?*

A: The cardinal sign that a caregiving plan isn't working and a
caregiver is in trouble is when physical violence occurs. I believe that, in
those situations, the caregiving plan must be immediately revised for the
protection of both the patient and caregiver, who each may be physically hurt but are certain to be psychologically damaged by such alterca-
tions. While it's understandable that pressures build and tempers flare,
safety has to be ensured. When tensions continue to lead to shaking,
slapping, hitting, kicking, or hair pulling, we can say that caregiving has
ceased to be caring and has become a source of mutual endangerment.

So, how can you restore a degree of safety? A first step is to arrange
for an immediate respite from caregiving. This is more easily said than
done, as you're probably aware. I'd try reaching out to family members
first to see if they can care for your mother for about a week so you can get
some rest and regain your composure. If family isn't willing or able and
you have sufficient money, you could consider hiring home health aides
to care for her in your home for several days. Depending on your
mother's age, there may be funding available through your county's Area
Agency on Aging to place her in a skilled nursing facility temporarily.
There's also a slim chance your mother's health insurance company
would agree to finance short-term respite services if, by doing so, it can
shore you up and then avoid having to pay (in part) for long-term
nursing home placement.

During this respite, it's crucial to meet with your family physician to
talk frankly about what has happened and what you've been feeling. He
or she is sure to discuss caregiver burnout with you and will probably also
evaluate you for major depression. Increased anger, heightened agitation, and decreased impulse control are common symptoms of that debilitating psychiatric disorder; taking an antidepressant or a mood-stabi-
lizing drug (such as Depakote) may help you get your feelings back under
control and allow you to manage your anger without lashing out physically. Counseling may also be of assistance to you to find better ways of
alleviating your frustrations with your mother. It's only when you feel
you can deal with your emotions better that you should consider
returning to caregiving.

In terms of your specific question about handling your emotions
when they're about to get the better of you, you may attempt the follow-

ing: Try to recall who your mother has been over your lifetime, not just the impaired, difficult woman she's become; the more you can allow yourself to empathize with her losses, the more your anger will be transformed into sadness and violence will be reduced. Try to remember who you've been—a person of love and dignity with a desire to help, not hurt, others. Identify those moments or interactions with your mother when tensions tend to be highest—for instance, toileting in the middle of the night or getting in and out of the car—and then devise specific plans for decreasing those tensions or, if that's not possible, refraining from inflaming each other. If you try these strategies and still are on the verge of shaking her at times, quickly remove yourself from those situations by going into another room, leaving the house for a walk around the block, or picking up the phone and ventilating to a friend. Those will be acts of kindness, not abandonment. If all else fails and violence persists, ceasing to provide care to your mother any longer and instead making other caregiving arrangements will be the kindest act of all.

CHAPTER FIVE

Weighing Hope and Acceptance, Fantasy and Reality

What exactly should they expect with Mother's cancer? After they attend the next appointment with her medical oncologist, neither sister is sure. The oncologist, a short, graying man in his late forties with a crisp lab coat and a formal air, treated them cordially but with tight-lipped caution. Mother asked few questions; he volunteered little information. When the sisters, with Mother's permission, asked to speak with him alone, he gave them a somber look and then led them from the exam room down the hall to a small carpeted office whose walls were covered with wooden-framed diplomas, glossy plaques, and family photographs. "Our mother doesn't want to know what's going to happen to her, but we do so we can plan better for the future," the older sister began. The oncologist cleared his throat and then slowly unreeled what sounded like a stock speech, citing research about people who seemed to have little to do with Mother and broad generalities about probable clinical scenarios. It was a fuzzy sketch when what the sisters wanted was a detailed tableau. The older sister, annoyed, felt compelled to try pressuring him. She kept saying, "I know you don't have a crystal ball . . ." before attempting to pin him down with specific questions. He responded by repeating the same generalities about the disease before finally saying in mild irritation, "Yes, I don't have a crystal ball. Few doctors do. We'll have to just wait and evaluate the response to the treatments." The sisters stopped asking questions, and the meeting wrapped up quickly. "I'm sure we'll have a chance to talk again," the doctor said, resuming his cordial tone as he walked them to the waiting room. The older sister replied with a curt "Yes" as she strode past him toward where her mother was slouched on a leather couch, an unopened women's magazine on her lap.

On the elevator down to the office building lobby, the sisters cast sympathetic glances at each other over their frustrations with the doctor's evasiveness. With eyes fixed on the elevator door in front of her, Mother seems to take no notice. Nor does she ask them about what her oncologist said. The younger daughter wants to say something reassuring to her, but Mother appears to be somewhere off in her own head. How could she not want to know what's going to happen to her?, the younger sister wonders. Is not knowing a way to remain positive or a kind of superstitious practice? Mother's own willful mother, the younger sister recalls, was an immigrant full of Old Country beliefs that talking about bad things made them more likely to happen, keeping mum less probable to occur. Perhaps subconsciously, under the current duress, Mother was reverting to her youth's lessons and embracing silence toward the cancerous threat. Speak no evil; hear no evil; suffer no evil.

As the elevator door opens and Mother shuffles out without looking at her daughters, the younger sister stares after her, unsure yet again whether she should leave her mother alone or try to get her to talk about what they're all facing. So what exactly are they facing? There's the question again. The doctor had talked about why further surgery was not indicated and chemotherapy was her best hope. He had described chemo's side effects, including fatigue, stomach upset, and possibly loss of hair. Mother's hair is thin anyway, the younger sister thinks. But the fact that he steered away from any talk about a prognosis—the question of what would happen—seems to her a bad sign. Doctors, she believes, don't like to rob patients and family members of all hope when the outlook is bleak. That's how they rationalize keeping them somewhat in the dark. Because we live in a litigious society, they probably also don't want to say anything for fear they'll be sued if they turn out to be wrong. Even if the family members ask directly about knowing everything, they hesitate. Even if someone as aggressive as her older sister is doing the asking, they bob and weave and stick to being vague.

Not that the younger sister wants all hope ripped from her. If the oncologist had said today, "I'm sorry, but your mother is going to be dead in 3 months," she would have collapsed right there on the thick carpet. It would have been impossible to look Mother in the face when she went out into the waiting room. It would be unthinkable to watch Doris Day movies with her mother anymore without continually choking back tears. But being left uncertain about the future doesn't exactly bolster her sense of optimism either. Whenever she encounters a vacuum of information, it's usually dread, not hope, that rushes in to fill the void. She has a vivid imagination for dire consequences. She could convince herself to expect the worst—for instance, Mother will experience crippling, unrelenting pain for which her daughters will be helpless to provide relief. At least if the doctor had spelled out some of the negative scenarios and dispelled some of the medical uncertainty, the younger sister's darkest imaginings might be held in check.

As they head down corridor after corridor toward the garage, the younger sister can see how uncertainty is affecting her sibling, too. Her older sister, when miffed, has always become vigorous in her movements. Bustling down the hallway now with quick, scuffling steps, she looks agitated. But because Mother can only toddle along, the older sister repeatedly stops and glances behind her with undisguised irritation as if scolding her mother to hurry up. The younger sister feels a surge of protective instinct toward the frail old woman and hurries to take Mother's arm in hers to buck her up. "Slow down a bit," the younger sister indignantly tells her sibling, who wheels around and stops with a fierce look but says nothing. "I'll drive Mom home," the younger sister continues. "No, I will," the older sister snaps at her. "Let me," the younger sister says just as insistently, "You seem stressed." Her older sister is about to retort again when Mother cuts in. "You know," she says in her own sharp tone, "I'm not too far gone to be asked to make my own choice. And I can't stand this stupid quibbling between the two of you."

Both daughters immediately go silent. It's as if this sick woman has been momentarily transformed into their domineering mother again and the two of them back into chastened children. The younger daughter looks abashed; the older one looks hurt and angry. The mother continues, turning toward her older child and saying in a kinder tone, "You're in a bad mood. Surely whatever my doctor told you can't be that bad." The older daughter grimaces and says, "The problem is he wouldn't tell us very much. He just gave us a lot of statistics and technical talk." "Don't be so sure that doctors know everything," Mother responds. "Besides, maybe there are things we're all better off not knowing."

The older daughter grunts in exasperation. The younger daughter shoots her a cross look before saying, "Come on, Mom. Let's get you home, and then we can talk." They start heading back down the hall at a slower pace but haven't gone more than 10 yards before the older daughter announces matter-of-factly, "I'm going to drive you home, Mother." The younger daughter decides just to give in to avoid further argument. Mother continues trudging ahead and says nothing but gives her younger daughter's arm a soft squeeze.

Most people cope best when they have a sense of control over what's going to happen to them. Divergent notions of what constitutes control, in fact, often account for differences in the ways patients and family members react to medical crises. Some individuals believe knowledge is power—a means of controlling their future health. They scour medical websites, join chat rooms, and compare multiple physicians' opinions to glean the treatment secrets, promising protocols, and alternative remedies for overcoming their serious ills.

Others find knowledge disempowering. Being on the receiving end of definitive medical pronouncements strips them of feeling any control over a disease's outcome and, consequently, their life course. When they attempt to shield themselves from or simply reject information, we call it "denial." Mother could have said, "Cancer? What cancer? Their test results don't make sense to me." When they attend to information selectively, we call it "minimization," more common than outright denial for maintaining control. Mother could say, "I know I have cancer, but the doctor said the chemo should do the trick. I'll be better in no time." People who find knowledge disempowering will downplay the physician's mention of possible failure or future recurrence to shunt it from awareness, at least temporarily.

Because the flow of medical information plays so large a part in the sense of control and well-being of some patients and family members, doctors are often treated like potential adversaries—either squeezed for more information or kept at arm's length to better deflect what they say. While experienced physicians expect these types of reactions and work toward accommodating the information preferences of patients and their relatives, many still find the whole exercise frustrating. I went into medicine to help people, they commonly complain, not to be pulled at or pushed away as if I'm part of their health problems.

Many have their own personal biases about whether patients and family members should be told every scrap of medical information or just given the CliffsNotes version or spared the gory details entirely. Some have qualms about sharing information with the patient's relatives, believing their job is to cure the sick member and not cater to his worried loved ones.

These various styles of handling information play out against the backdrop of a shifting medical culture. Forty years ago old-time paternalism reigned. Doctors thought of themselves as the experts not only on disease but on what patients should be told about their conditions and when—an authoritative role later maligned as "playing God." The most notorious example of this was the not infrequent practice of withholding the distressing news that a patient had cancer for fear that the knowledge would demoralize him and thereby hasten his death.

But as American culture has become more open and inclusive, so has medicine over the past three decades. The ideal physician–patient relationship, say the current medical textbooks and consumer health guides, is one of partnership. Patients now maintain a sense of control by assuming the role of customers who purchase medical services and therefore have a right to know all the details of every intervention, much the way an owner has a right to the whys and wherefores of the repair of her automobile. For those patients who don't want to know—for whom denial or minimization serves as a coping mechanism because complete disclosure would overwhelm them—physician-partners are supposed to comply by supplying only the amount of information desired. For example, the American Medical Association widely disseminated a training module on "End-of-Life Care" in 2000 that advises doctors to ask patients and family members how much they want to know before communicating bad news.

Most of the time, the spirit of partnership works; patients, relatives, and healthcare professionals pull together in a coordinated attack on the disease. When, on occasion, the partnerships don't coalesce into effective working units, it's generally because there are mismatches between the communication styles or information-sharing preferences of particular patients and physicians. A mistrustful patient and a bold physician often don't mix well. Neither do a frightened patient and a close-to-the-vest physician. When the personalities of specific family members are factored in—for instance, when a pushy relative expresses uninformed and unsolicited opinions to both patient and doctor about medical issues—the partnership is even more strained. It's at those moments that patients and family members are prone to seeking control over their circumstances in another way—breaking ranks with their doctors and blaming them for all that goes wrong medically. At those times physicians and nurses are likely to retaliate, griping to one another about their "difficult" patients with their "manipulative" or "intrusive" relatives who are "getting in the way of treatment."

When the partnerships break down, the patient's prognosis is often one of the main areas of disagreement. Stakes are high here; few questions matter more to gaining a sense of control than what the disease's course is likely to be. Typically, healthcare professionals, drawing on their scientific knowledge and clinical experience, take a more circumspect view than do patients and relatives, who put greater faith in the patient's will to live, the hand of God, and the healing power of family and community support. Sometimes, though, it's the professionals who put so much credence in biomedical technologies that they want to keep fighting the disease long after the patient and family members have become resigned to the likelihood of death. (It's like the old joke commonly told in hospice organizations: Question: Why are there nails in coffins? Answer: To keep the medical oncologist out.) In both these scenarios, it's difficult to tell which attitudes reflect reasonable hope—essential for keeping up morale—and which are sheer fantasy—well-intended but pie-in-the-sky wishfulness. Not only do professionals, patients, and their family members disagree on what to expect; among patients and their relatives, there are often sharp disagreements about whose vision of the future should hold sway. If one family member seems overly pessimistic, then the others may debate him vociferously. If another seems overly optimistic, then others may make comments to bring him down to earth. As the medical crisis drags on, the tension between hope and fantasy often increases and becomes a major stressor for everyone involved.

The tension between hope and fantasy occurs within each individual family member and often between family members. Are you largely optimistic or pessimistic? What about your relatives? Do differences among you cause conflicts when caregiving and medical decisions have to be made?

Lying once more in her granddaughter's old room, staring at the yellowing posters on the walls and the discolored troll dolls atop the nicked dresser, the mother feels like she's been thrust back in time more than 6 weeks. Then she had been laid up here with abdominal pain from her hysterectomy. Now she's convalescing with stultifying fatigue. Since starting the chemotherapy, her body feels sheathed in lead. Her head feels to her like a cannon ball pulling down her neck. Even her eyes feel too heavy to open, as if she's already dead and silver dollars have been placed on her lids. Before the chemo, the mother felt old and gray; now she feels ancient and drained of all color. After rolling over in bed and carefully creeping over to the commode, she's completely exhausted for a half-hour. Trying to yell downstairs for her daughter to take away her untouched bowl of broth, she's appalled at how her voice weakly croaks.

This isn't what she wanted. During the first week of the treatments, when her younger daughter was driving her several mornings a week to the hospital's chemotherapy suite, Mother had insisted on staying in her own apartment. But after only a few days she noticed her feet were dragging slowly across the carpet. Then one afternoon, leaning on the back of the couch as she maneuvered in the living room, her legs suddenly gave way and she fell hard on her shoulder and head. More stunned than hurt, she lay there for 20 minutes, unable to rise, before she remembered the cell phone that her children had forced her to carry. She called her older daughter, who left work immediately. Racing into the apartment 45 minutes later to find her mother looking dazed on the couch, the daughter blurted "I'm calling the doctor!" before even asking how the old woman was. A 3-hour wait in the emergency room and a set of CT scans and other tests later, it was concluded that Mother had not broken anything, suffered a heart attack, or had any internal bleeding but should probably not stay alone. By dinnertime, the daughters had deposited her with a valise full of house clothes and toiletries back into the granddaughter's room. Mother had been too tired and ashamed to protest.

In the week since then, the mother has received assurances from her internist that her lack of energy is a byproduct of the chemotherapy and not a sign that her cancer is worsening. But with each day she spends struggling to lift her head from her pillow, she becomes more convinced she has had a major setback. It's not necessarily a medical setback, however (though, she recalls, when her husband's cancer was spreading steadily, his doctors also swore that his disease was in remission). In her mind, it's more a relapse of fortune. The fact that something bad has happened to her, regardless of its reason, is evidence that more bad things are likely to occur. Whatever assumptions she had made that everything was going to turn out all right have been punctured. Whatever prayers she prayed now seem for naught. She realizes she's an old woman, sick and extremely tired. She learned long ago that life takes its own course in its own time. If it's her turn to head downhill, how can she possibly try to reverse that momentum?

In the past few days she's watched her daughter observing her whenever she scurries into the room with folded laundry and pitchers of ice water. (The oncologist had suggested keeping Mother hydrated; the daughter is filling her to the gills.) While scrutinizing her closely, the daughter wears a slight frown as if she doesn't like what she sees. Seeing that telltale frown, Mother believes her daughter probably thinks she's depressed. But Mother herself feels depression isn't what she's experiencing. What she's experiencing is resignation. Sure, she'll try as hard as she can to get strong and well, but she's willing to accept whatever comes. If she tries explaining that to her older daughter, however, she'll get nowhere; her daughter will react instantly with strong disdain that her mother is selfishly giving up. It's as if the mother is supposed to fight for her daughter's sake as well as her own. It's as though she'll be personally letting her daughter down if, through some wavering of her will, she happens to succumb to the disease. So, the two of them don't talk much about Mother's morale because the old woman sees nothing productive coming out of it. Instead, when the daughter looks at her hard, Mother gazes back with as much cheerfulness as her fatigue will allow as a way of showing her daughter she's really okay. The problem is, the older daughter returns Mother's cheery look with raised eyebrows indicating skepticism and a deepening frown signaling concern.

The past few months have been highly vexing for the older daughter. Worried about her mother's well-being, she has rearranged her life to do whatever has been necessary to care for her. Her husband has hardly seen her. She missed her grandkids' recent recitals and soccer games. She took a leave from work precipitously, then returned to it briefly until, mere weeks later, she had to take another sudden leave; it's a wonder her employer is bearing with her. None of these sacrifices, however, has been too much. But what she finds intolerable is that, while she does all she can to give her mom the best fighting chance, her mother seems to be frittering away her natural tenacity. Mother was always the ferociously tough one in the family; it was her father and younger sister who moped when stressed. It's beyond the older daughter's comprehension why cancer or its treatments should transform who her mother has always been. The listless woman who's lying in the upstairs bed is practically unrecognizable to her. Yes, she sympathizes with the fact that chemo has taken the starch out of her. But the look in her mother's eyes isn't the determined look of a fighter anymore.

This isn't just a sentimental matter. While she's aware it would be unrealistic to expect her mother to be the tigress of her youth, all she's ever heard about cancer is that hope and staying positive are weapons as important as chemo and radiation. If Mother becomes complacent or, worse, throws in the towel, she may be signing her own death certificate. The older daughter isn't ready to lose her mother. Therefore, she must do all she can to bring about a turnaround in Mother's attitude.

There's little use in appealing to her mother's physicians for help with this, the older daughter tells herself. In the old days, she believes, doctors used to specialize in inspiring hope. They knew just what to say to lift your spirits and wouldn't hang crepe until the very end. But now doctors are too worried about being sued to risk saying anything they can't predict with absolute surety. Her mother's oncologist, she thinks, is an aloof prig who won't dare speak his mind. Her internist is warmer and more accommodating but is in such a rush he doesn't have the time to tell you anything. They don't generate hope; they evoke uncertainty.

Then there's her sensitive sister, the older daughter reflects sarcastically. She comes several days a week to spend an hour sitting by Mother's bed, practically lapping up every gripe she utters. It's almost as if the younger daughter encourages their mother's pessimism; it's as if they're wallowing together in negative "stinking thinking." As far as the older daughter is concerned, that's not inspiring hope either—it's strangling it. For her sake, Mother needs to be directed to keep her mind on the positive. If necessary, the older daughter is prepared to confront her sister about adopting a more upbeat stance.

The younger daughter senses the stiffness in her sister's manner each time she stops in the kitchen on the way upstairs to visit Mother. She's unsure why until her older sibling makes a snide comment one day that "Mother seems to enjoy crying to you." While her first impulse is to react defensively, she has a sudden insight about what's going on. Her older sister has never tolerated sadness very well, preferring cheers to tears. She probably wants her to give Mother a bracing pep talk to snap her out of her torpor. But the younger daughter has never been comfortable with fantasies. She prefers reality straight up, however grim. In her mind, there's no making the mother's fatigue vanish with chest thumping or happy talk. There's no sugarcoating the rigors of cancer. What her mother needs, she believes, is someone to listen to whatever she's feeling, not try to persuade her to feel differently. Rather than debating her older sister, the younger daughter just shrugs her shoulders, turns around, and continues on upstairs without comment. She will not be deterred by her from doing what she thinks is best.

There's something in particular that, for the past few days, she has been thinking may be for the best. Perhaps the chemo is too much for Mother. Perhaps a respite is in order until she can regain some strength. She hasn't yet raised this possibility with her. Such a plan would have to be cleared with the oncologist, and there's no telling how he'd react. The older daughter would also have to be on board, or Mother would never agree without fearing that she was letting her down. Her sister would likely balk at the idea, arguing that Mother needs to keep fighting. She might even become incensed at the very notion of a respite. Then the younger daughter would really have a battle on her hands. But, for the mother's sake, she still feels the subject has to be broached.

Reentering the kitchen after descending the stairs, the younger daughter glances quickly at her sister, who's sitting sullenly at the table and then averts her eyes. She makes no introductory comments but gets right to the point. "The chemo is too much for her," she says in a quiet but firm voice. "She needs a break from it. Maybe for a few weeks or a month." The older daughter opens her mouth to respond, then closes it again as if forcefully stifling something she was about to say. The younger daughter sits down on the other side of the table and waits for her sister to answer. The older daughter twists in her chair and then places her hands, palms down, carefully on the table in front of her. "We are not on the same page," she says in an uncharacteristically low voice. "We are working at cross-purposes. I only want to keep Mom's hope alive—to keep her alive—and you keep dragging her down. If she quits the treatment, there's no telling whether she'll have enough confidence to go back to it. She has to believe it's going to help her. But you'll convince her it's harmful to her."

The younger sister takes this in silently. There's a long pause before she finally responds, "I don't know if the treatment is helping kill the cancer or not. I do know it's wiping her out. I'm all for increasing hope, but I don't want to create any fantasies that, if she just hangs in there with this horrible chemo, she'll be fine. You'd like to make her think she's going to be fine, but she may just suffer more."

The older sister doesn't respond. The two of them stare at each other's hands on the tabletop. After a few moments, the younger sister finally asks, "Why don't we bring it up with the oncologist before we decide whether or not to present it as an option to Mom? Let's get his opinion."

The older sister exhales loudly and says with thick sarcasm, "We had such a productive meeting with him last time." The younger sister pauses again before saying quietly, "I'll go without you if I have to. I'm going to ask him." Her sister says nothing but stares at her stonily. She then pushes herself away from the table and slowly walks out of the room.

"The power of positive thinking," once the title of a best-selling popular psychology book, is also a commonly held belief in our culture. We talk about silver linings and the darkness before the dawn. We reach for the stars while keeping our chins up because hope springs eternal. The entire American ethos of pushing into new frontiers is based on the supposition that we have within us the determination to face all challenges and succeed.

Within academic circles, there has been substantial research over the past two decades on the positive impact of positive attitudes and beliefs. In the late 1980s and early 1990s, social psychologists Shelley E. Taylor and Jonathon D. Brown wrote extensively about the beneficial effects of "positive illusions." They concluded that when people believe in themselves and their capabilities for dealing with untoward events, regardless of their actual ability to handle them, they cope much better overall. In other words, overrating yourself frequently helps. Or, conversely, if you regard yourself and your environment more realistically, you may be less able to cope and more prone to depression. Brown theorized that illusions work in several ways. If you believe you're hot stuff, then you're more likely to judge negative circumstances as challenging rather than crushing. If you believe that you've got what it takes to rise to any occasion, then you'll take actions with confidence rather than remain passive in fear. If you confidently take action, then you'll feel greater control over adverse situations and therefore have less emotional distress.

During the 1990s and 2000s, a "positive psychology" movement has also spread widely. Led by University of Pennsylvania psychologist Martin Seligman, researchers from a variety of disciplines have studied how the ways people explain life events to themselves shape their emotional reactions to those events. A touchstone of the movement is the finding that when people are raised to be optimistic—retaining positive beliefs about the future even during difficult times—they contend better with life's catastrophes without falling into depression. When they develop explanatory styles that lead them toward pessimistic outlooks and self-blame, they stumble more frequently into despair.

Applying the theories of positive illusions and positive psychology to cancer care, we can surmise that believing you're going to beat the disease has advantages over being consumed with anxiety about your fate. You may regard typical treatment complications as bumps in the road, not the end of the line. You may muster the strength to advocate for yourself rather than allow others to dictate what's going to happen to you. If you're a caregiver, your faith that you're fighting a winnable battle may be a balm to your fatigue and self-sacrifice.

But questions remain about whether positivity works for all people across the range of possible tragedies. Life-altering illness is a tough circumstance in which to hold to an unwavering posture. At such times optimism about the patient's treatments can serve as a shield for people against the assault of demoralizing prognoses. Even in the sad event that a loved one's disease proves fatal, an optimistic belief among relatives that the family will somehow survive may protect them all from feeling lost. But unmitigated optimism can also be a blindfold. Worn too tightly, it may block patients and their loved ones from really seeing and responding to the dangerous straits they're in. It's at those times that healthcare professionals, when complaining about those they serve, start throwing around damning putdowns such as "They're in denial." Seligman himself wrote at the end of his popular book *Learned Optimism* that "Optimism is no panacea." No amount of hope can negate reality. Refusing to accept the vicissitudes of an illness is no positive achievement; it's a strategy that will hinder, not aid, long-term psychological adjustment.

So, how should family caregivers and their ill loved ones weigh hope and acceptance, fantasy and reality? Revisiting the popular metaphor about the cup of water—in which optimists see it as half-full and pessimists as half-empty—can help guide us. Perceiving the glass as three-quarters empty when the volume in actuality is at least a quarter higher is a distortion of reality that we commonly associate with depression. It will make illness's consequences feel more painful; it will increase suffering. By the same token, perceiving the glass as three-quarters full when the volume is actually a quarter lower is a distortion of reality we associate with Pollyannaish delusions. It substitutes naive belief for preparedness; it makes any negative outcomes of illness more shocking and excruciating. Both types of distortions should be guarded against.

But when it comes to the age-old debate between half-empty and half-full, it's not a matter of avoiding equally harmful distortions; it's a task of weighing the potential benefits of more or less reality-based perceptions. And on this the research is clear: Half-full works better. (Even seeing it as a little more than half—say, two-thirds full—is stretching reality slightly but is generally okay.) Reasonably optimistic patients and their family members strive harder to find the best treatments. When they believe they've found them, they follow them with all the more rigor. Hope carries them through rough patches. Staying positive allows them to try new solutions when the ones in place aren't effective. Being optimistic shouldn't preclude having feelings of worry or anger or sadness. The squelching of those feelings because they're too "negative" can itself be damaging. But the feelings shouldn't undermine a basic belief that everything will likely work out in the end: The illness will be managed, the family will go on. Patients and caregivers and professionals should all be united to fight this good fight. They should fight it believing they'll ultimately, if arduously, prevail. There's nothing fancy or innovative about these strategies; most of us commonly refer to them as being cautiously optimistic (with an emphasis on the cautiousness).

Cautious optimism means . . .

- Holding on to enough hope to keep fighting the good fight while maintaining a firm enough grip on reality to see what's happening and respond appropriately to changing needs.
- Keeping the daily ups and downs in perspective and your emotional reactions to them under control.
- Avoiding being so inflexibly positive that you blind yourself to real dangers and jeopardize the physician–patient–caregiver partnership.

So, how do you find the balance we call cautious optimism in your own battle against serious illness? The first step is to be aware of all you know about the disease and the patient to try to judge the medical situation as realistically as possible. You can't easily manage this first step, however, without mastering two others: Try to avoid the roller coaster of emotional reactions to every new development in your loved one's condition. In other words, when prognostic signs on a given day are good, don't conclude that a cure is at hand. When signs are bad, don't count the patient out. A third step is to let time pass, events unfold, and emotions settle. The longer, more dispassionate view of the situation you take will be the most accurate. You'll then be in a better position to assume a stance that's sensibly optimistic without being willfully foolish.

Back in the oncologist's office, the sisters sit alone in the chrome-and-rattan armchairs in front of the black lacquer desk, reading the diplomas and awards on the walls as they wait for Mother's doctor to finish up an "important phone call." They can actually hear the oncologist's muffled voice coming through the wall from an adjoining office. Although they cannot make out his words, they can hear his deep, sober monotone and measured rhythms. He sounds every bit the serious, self-controlled technician. When they hear him emit a short, percussive guffaw at one point, the two sisters look at each other with smirks as if each is surprised to hear that the man is capable of a human response. A moment later, a second thought goes through the older daughter's mind—Why is this guy laughing while letting us wait in here for 20 minutes?—and the smirk disappears from her face. She had disagreed with her sister about even setting up this meeting and then had found herself unable to resist attending it for fear of being left out. Now she's impatient to get on with it and go home.

A few minutes later, the oncologist enters the room, shakes their hands briskly, and slips into the black leather chair behind the desk. As the younger daughter expresses her concerns about how the chemotherapy has sapped her mother of all strength, he listens with a neutral expression, occasionally jotting notes on a legal pad. He remains impassive when the younger daughter asks, "Would it make sense for Mother to take a break from the chemotherapy?" But when the older daughter jumps in, asking "What harm could it cause her?" before he has a chance to address the first question, he puts down his pen and frowns slightly for the first time.

"It all depends," he says in a straightforward professional tone. "The available research suggests that a short respite won't change the outcome of her treatment. But these are only probabilities. It may affect your mother differently." The younger daughter stares at him and blinks. The older daughter grits her teeth. She doesn't want to hear about research; she wants to be told what he thinks they should do. The oncologist seems to sense her disgruntlement, because he suddenly shifts in his seat and says more rapidly, "A break in treatment is advisable if she's so debilitated. The risks are likely small."

"Oh, good," says the younger daughter. "I'm glad to hear that. She's been suffering. I'm sure she'll be glad to hear that, too." The older daughter says nothing but stares straight ahead at the physician.

"But," the oncologist continues with greater emphasis, "I'd like to keep the stoppage short. The treatment is essential." There's a pause before the older daughter responds, "Of course." The younger daughter then asks in a small voice, "Is it really essential?"

The oncologist eyes her closely as if trying to perceive her meaning. "I don't quite grasp your question," he says, perplexed. "I mean," says the younger daughter hastily as if feeling defensive, "will the drug really help?"

The oncologist's eyes widen as if sensing his judgment is being challenged. "It's the gold standard for this type of cancer," he says with a hint of exasperation. "It's not just some pipe dream so we feel like we're doing something. Its track record is generally fair."

"She's not talking about the drug," interjects the older daughter. "She's wondering if it's worth putting Mother through this chemo or any other treatment you can come up with if she's just going to die anyway."

The younger daughter glances at her sister, then looks down in embarrassment before turning her eyes back to the physician. The oncologist says "Oh" before shifting again in his seat and pushing his legal pad off to the side of the desk. The older daughter is wondering if he's going to get angry or just quote more statistics at them. Instead, he says to the two sisters in a softer voice than they've heard him use: "I can understand how frightening and distressing this all is for the two of you. I've been through this kind of thing in my own family. I deal with this in my work life every day. You may not believe it, but these are no longer the bad old days when a cancer diagnosis was an absolute death knell. We've made advances; there are things to be hopeful about. Your mother has possibilities to be hopeful about."

He looks at the younger daughter, who gazes back steadily. Rather than looking heartened by what he's just said, she looks dejected. The older daughter, in contrast, looks surprised and impressed. "If you don't approach this with some positive sense, then the treatments aren't going to be as effective," he says gently to the younger daughter. "Your mother will pick up on your discouragement, and part of her will give up. I can't guarantee exactly how well your mother will do once she goes back on the chemotherapy, but I can tell you that without hope she won't have much future. Do you understand what I'm getting at?"

The younger daughter answers, "Yes. You want me to give treatment a fair chance. You think my attitude will affect my mother's." "That's right," the oncologist answers. "Your optimism will support hers. She really does need hope to keep going." He pauses briefly before continuing, "Consider this a pep talk. Anytime you need another one, let me know." As they stand up and head toward the door, the oncologist adds: "Unless I can maintain an attitude that's realistic and positive, I could never do my job. I'd have thrown up my hands within a month of completing my training. We all need hope."

When they step into the elevator, the younger daughter says immediately, "Don't ever put me on the spot again by telling him I'm questioning all treatment." Her sister responds, "That's fine so long as you stop counting Mom out before she's gone. I'm not going to put up with it." The younger daughter has the impulse to argue with her but thinks better of it. A moment later, she answers simply, "I'll try."

Finding the means to stay hopeful while avoiding subscribing to fantasies about your loved one's illness is a difficult but crucial balance to strike. As preferable as fantasies are to contemplating the devastation that disease can bring, they can blind you to unpleasant realities for which you must prepare. The balances between hope and acceptance, reality and fantasy, must be constantly revised as the illness progresses and conditions shift. Not everyone makes these shifts easily, though. Many caregivers, once perspectives and routines are established, are resistant to giving them up. In the next chapter, we will discuss the prerequisite for achieving those revisions as change unfolds—a capacity for maintaining awareness and flexibility.

Bucking the Family Tide of Denial

Q: *I come from a reserved family in which nobody likes to talk about any bad news. I think they're all in denial most of the time. When my grand-*

mother was dying of congestive heart failure, everyone made believe she'd be as good as new after a short hospitalization. They just got angry when the doctors tried to tell them otherwise. They got furious with me when I tried to raise the possibility that Grams might not make it. After she died, they all commiserated together but made me feel like a bad guy. How do I handle this?

A: The common expression "Don't shoot the messenger" sums it up perfectly. Most of us try to deflect bad news. When it's forced on us anyway, we tend to get angry, not at the grim tidings, but at the person conveying them. Being the messenger is generally an unenviable role to play in a family, even if you think it's your duty to pull everyone's head out of the sand for their own good.

I don't think confronting your family members is necessarily the best way to get through to them. They'll likely just feel attacked, not enlightened, and reject what you say out of hand. Sowing the seeds of later understanding is usually a more effective approach, though one that demands great patience. I'd suggest sharing all available medical information with them and pointing out your close observations of the patient without drawing any prognostic conclusions. It's essential to restrain yourself from reacting when they pooh-pooh your concerns; if you argue with them, they'll just smirk and dismiss you as an alarmist. Over time, as the patient begins failing and they hear more bad news from the medical team, they'll start making their own observations rather than simply relying on their beliefs. Even with blinders on, they'll see more of what is happening and arrive at their own conclusions. In all probability, reality will slowly sink in.

Another factor to consider is what psychologists call "groupthink." Family members in a group setting, such as a family meeting or holiday dinner, are more likely to adhere loyally to the family line on the patient's illness—for example, "She'll be fine." But the same relatives when approached as individuals, away from the strong influence of other members, will be more likely to entertain other perspectives, even a pessimistic one. With that in mind, you'll probably have more luck convincing others of your viewpoint if you talk with each of them one-on-one.

A third strategy involves focusing on the one or two leaders in the family whose opinions weigh most heavily in all of the clan's decisions. If you can sway the patriarch or matriarch to prepare for dire possibilities, other family members may broaden their outlooks to take into account the prospect of a bad medical outcome.

The key in all these strategies is to avoid trying to overpower the group's denial. Family members need to protect one another by keeping reality at bay at times. So long as this doesn't prevent them from preparing for negative and positive outcomes as the patient declines, you should give your message gently and strategically out of respect for their beliefs.

Who Decides Whether Truth Is Cruel or Kind?

Q: *My father's doctor won't be straight with him about his cancer. She doesn't come right out and tell him that his chances of survival are small. Instead, she lets Dad delude himself into believing he's going to be all right. It strikes me as cruel. It also puts me in the position of having to put a damper on my father's unrealistic expectations—my mother died several years ago, and now everything is up to me. How can I get the doctor to stop feeding my father's fantasies?*

A: A good first step would be to try to understand why the doctor behaves as she does. Several possibilities exist. She may believe that keeping your father in the dark will preserve his hope and buoy his spirits at a bleak time in his life. She may have asked your father how much he wants to know—as American Medical Association end-of-life guidelines recommend—and your father told her he doesn't want to hear the prognosis. Or perhaps the physician has had personal experiences—for instance, the death of one of her own family members from cancer—that make her loath to discuss such issues with her patients. It's incumbent upon you to initiate a dialogue with her (while your father is not present) to find out her guiding philosophy. During that discussion, you can explain to her the ramifications for you and the rest of the family of her relative lack of communication.

An important second step is to reflect on whether it is, in fact, cruel for your father to be unaware of his prognosis. While we all will face death one day, most of us wouldn't choose to live with an awareness of a sword hanging over our heads. If not knowing that his chances of survival are poor allows him to focus on living rather than dying during his time remaining, then keeping him ignorant may be wise. The best judge of this, however, is your father. I'd suggest asking him how much he wants to know and then respecting those wishes.

Finally, it would serve you well through this very difficult time to reflect on your own attitudes about approaching death with full understanding. Have you had previous experiences in which a loved one suffered from ignorance that have convinced you your father needs to be cognizant of all that will happen? Do you want him to know his chances are slim so the two of you can grieve together while there's still time? By better grasping your own reactions and motives here, you can negotiate a common understanding with the doctor and your father of how much reality is just enough.

The Car Keys: Emblem of Independence

Q: *My father, who suffers from a progressive neurological disorder, has been in a wheelchair for many years but continued to drive to work until recently. After a minor mishap behind the wheel, he voluntarily decided to give up his car keys. Aside from the challenge of having to find alternative transportation for him, I'm dealing with the emotional toll that losing his independence has had on him, and me. He has always been there for me while I've been raising a young son alone. How do I help him cope with the pain of making this courageous decision, and how do I deal with this further reminder that all of our lives will get harder and harder?*

A: With each inevitable downturn in the progression of a neurological disorder—from quick wits to scrambled thought, from sturdy legs to stair glides—there's a sense of painful loss. But nothing makes people feel like their grip has slipped from the steering wheel of their own lives more than losing the privilege to drive. Particularly for men, it's a threshold that, once crossed, makes them feel they've lost not only their independence but, to a degree, themselves. It's little wonder they frequently fight it long past the point of being able to competently handle an automobile. Often the car keys have to be literally wrested from them. Your father is to be commended for realizing his increasing limitations and putting others' safety above his need to remain behind the wheel.

In truth, there are no easy answers to your wrenching questions. Your life as a family has changed irreparably. Your lives will change yet more, irrevocably. Anger and sadness are the normal and expectable responses. To manage these emotions in order to prevent them from making misery out of what life you still share, here are some possibilities:

• One advantage of dealing with a progressive, rather than sudden, illness is that you have some time to anticipate and prepare for the declines in functioning that are coming. While such preparation may not make the losses any less sad when they occur, they generally help avoid the sharp sting of shock. Allow yourself and your father to fully grieve his recent loss of the ability to drive, brainstorm how you'll keep him as mobile and independent as possible—and then begin talking about what tragedy is coming down the pike next and how you'll cope with it. If the disease is unremitting, you have to be all the more proactive, brave, and cunning.

• Even if your father can no longer operate a motor vehicle, he must strive to be the driver of his own life. Make sure he retains as much decision-making power over where he goes and what he does as possible. As the Serenity Prayer says, let him control what he can, not continuously chafe about what he can't control. He may yet preserve parts of himself against his disease's marauding destruction.

• For some remarkably adaptable sufferers of neurological decline, the shift from riding in the driver's seat to the passenger's seat in life is merely one of perspective. They're still able to enjoy the scenery seen through the window in front of them rather than dwelling on where they're sitting or whether they're in control of the speed of the car. They're able to accept the services of a chauffeur—or a devoted daughter—without feeling like they're just bulk freight. They may even savor the ride all the more because it's now one shared with someone they cherish or love. For most of us, achieving such acceptance and equanimity is very difficult. But it may be what you and your father would do best to aim for as you ride out the long course together.

When Sadness Comes Out as Anger

Q: *My 78-year-old brother suffered a series of strokes and recently spent the last 4 months in a rehabilitation hospital near where his only daughter lives. I'm 15 years younger than my brother and have spent the past couple of years traveling some distance every few weeks to help care for my brother even though I have my own health problems. My niece has never gotten along with her father and plans to place him in an assisted living facility so far away that it will be impossible for me to continue to see him. I believe she's bitter that I'm listed as the only other beneficiary in my brother's will and is withholding information from me. She has stolen money from my brother, and I don't believe she has his best interests at heart. What can I do?*

A: In an ideal world, medical and psychiatric crises would bring family members together for the three Cs—commiseration, coordination of caregiving, and comforting the afflicted. In real life, however, such crises sometimes inflame relationships that have long been marred by emotional distance or chronic conflict. Relatives may struggle over who has the power to make decisions for the patient. They may gripe behind one another's back about who hasn't done his share of caregiving. They may balk at doing more. As the patient's condition spirals downward, tensions escalate. If and when the patient dies, the family's relationships may be fraught with greater antagonism than ever.

You seem to be caught up in the resentments and spitefulness of this type of caregiving family. Before you can decide the nature of the commitment you'd like to make to taking care of your brother, there are legal and psychological issues that are necessary to consider for your sake and your brother's.

The foremost legal issue is whether your brother has been deemed by a doctor to be competent to make decisions on his own behalf. If so, he has the right to choose where he'll live, how to spend his money, and the like, regardless of whether his daughter was previously designated his power of attorney or opposes his judgments. Your brother could even decide to live with you and cut his daughter out of the picture altogether. However, if a court, on the basis of his psychiatric evaluation, has declared your brother incompetent because of cognitive deficits following his stroke, your niece may have the power to make virtually all major decisions and withhold information from whomever she chooses. You'll then have to decide to fight against her or appeal to her.

Fighting would be difficult and risky. It's one thing for you to feel sure that your niece is trampling her father's best interests and pilfering his money. It's quite another for you to hire a lawyer to petition a court on those grounds in order to wrest guardianship away from your niece. Such cases require a heavy burden of proof. Even if a judge agrees with you, he or she would likely appoint a neutral *guardian ad litem* to oversee your brother's affairs; there's no telling whether that person would regard your interest in your brother favorably or not. The risk with taking any legal action, of course, is that you would essentially be declaring open warfare on your niece. If you lose, she'd have the power plus the incentive to punish you by limiting your contact with your brother even more than she already has.

Appealing to your niece with olive branch extended has certain psychological advantages. By conveying respect for her power, you stand a better chance of forging a more cordial and mutually beneficial working arrangement with her and then putting your commitment to your brother into operation. You never have to like or agree with her; you merely have to demonstrate that you're no threat to her in order to be included in the loop. I daresay your brother would be more comfortable if his two closest living relatives cooperated more. Otherwise he'd be caught in a loyalty bind between the two of you, ever sensitive to what you each may say about the other and probably never completely open about his own feelings with either of you. That would only compound any emotional problems stemming from his debilitation.

But the most important psychological reason for reaching out to your niece is that anger is often a cover for sadness. So long as the two of you dicker over control, you avoid mourning your brother's decline. Allowing yourselves to be sad together now will promote acceptance and make more bearable your brother's eventual death.

CHAPTER SIX

---∞---

Fostering Awareness and Flexibility

"**P**lease come down and try to help me," the older sister calls upstairs to the mother. She's trying to sound inviting, but there's a trace of testiness in her tone. For the first time in months, she's entertaining guests, and she's feeling pressured even though it's only family. She waits at the bottom of the stairs, listening to hear if Mother is rising from her bed. When, in a few moments, she doesn't detect the squeak of bedsprings or clomp of the walker, she turns on her heel and strides into the kitchen, figuring she'll have to chop all the vegetables herself.

Her husband and children had convinced her to have the whole family over for a big dinner to celebrate Mother's birthday. We don't know how many more she'll have, they reasoned. But in the older sister's mind, the more important cause for celebration is the end of Mother's chemo. Ten weeks of three-times-a-week treatment (interrupted early on by a week's respite) thankfully finished several days before. There would be no more futile searches for parking spots in the hospital garage, no more black-and-blue arm bruises from the IVs, no more complaints of crushing fatigue. The older sister would like to think it was also the end of Mother's cancer, but she's already been warned that it's too soon to declare that. The oncologist did his dry, conservative best to temper her hopes by reminding her that cancer is considered to be in remission only when no recurrence has been detected after 5 years. Five years, snorts the older sister. Mother could well be dead from old age by then. So the older sister has set her own measure for determining her mother's status: If the full-body CT scans planned for 2 months after her last chemo treatment show no more tumors or suspicious lesions, Mother has beaten her cancer—at least for the time being.

Lying motionless in a dreamy state, the mother is startled into alertness by her daughter's call but doesn't budge until she hears the daughter's footsteps heading away. Though still prone in bed, she's now tense with conflicting feelings. Part of her wants to hurry straightaway to the kitchen. She was the proud matriarch; for decades, she took charge of the family dinners at her house and, later, apartment without needing assistance from anybody. Even taking on a mere child's job today, such as cutting vegetables or setting the table, would be a small step toward recouping her natural position. But another part of her also resents even being asked to help. Why doesn't anyone see she's still tired? she carps to herself. Why can't an old lady simply rest on her birthday? Besides, the evening's festivities hold no great joy for her. Another year older at her age is no accomplishment; it's a liability. Later, she'll go through the motions of hugging her granddaughters and cooing to their babies while delivering the expected compliments. Her mind, however, will not be focused on the family's future generation but on its past. Thoughts of her husband, her own mother, and others who have departed will preoccupy her, as they have for several months. Surveying her daughter's crowded table, set with her own antique china, matching gilt-edged gravy boat, and fluted silverware, she'll be lost in visions of other family dinners from 40 or 50 years ago, when she was young and healthy and brimming with the kind of energy she lacks now.

As the mother clutches the banister and goes slowly down the stairs a step at a time, the older sister suddenly appears at the bottom of the staircase, arms akimbo, looking up with a mixture of judgment and concern. "Careful," she says sharply, then checks herself and says more softly, "Shall I come up and take your arm?" The mother keeps her eyes fixed on the next step downward and answers plainly, "No." When she reaches the first-floor landing and turns toward the kitchen, the older sister says, "I've already chopped most of the vegetables. Your favorite granddaughter will be here soon. Why don't you sit in the living room and wait for her?"

The mother sits alone for a half-hour in a deep, high-backed arm-chair. The older sister can be heard clanking pans and slamming cup-board doors in the kitchen. Like many people's living rooms, this room feels like more of a showcase for tasteful, heavy furniture than a place where loving people congregate. The air smells of lemon wood polish, and the yellowish light is dim. Mother has the ridiculous feeling of having been put out to pasture in this pristine space. Or, worse, she feels placed here as another family heirloom, more antiquated than valuable, for the great-grandchildren to stare at and hear tales of. Just then the doorbell rings, and the older sister bustles from the kitchen toward the front hallway. Her eldest daughter, trailed by a gangly hus-band and two young children, has arrived.

There's a round of kissing and hugging by the front door. The older sister stashes their coats in the closet and then leads them into the liv-ing room, where they line up to give the family matriarch swift pecks on her cool cheek. The aroma of roasting turkey and cooked carrots draws their attention to the kitchen. The older sister asks her grand-children, a 7-year-old boy and a 5-year-old girl, to help her stir the gravy, and they go dashing off. The gangly husband follows after them to help. The favorite granddaughter takes a seat on the floral-patterned couch by the armchair to have a talk with her ailing grandmother.

Sitting tall on the edge of the couch, the granddaughter has her fa-ther's erect posture but her mother's matronly girth; two pregnancies before age 30 have expanded her once girlish figure. From her mother and grandmother, she's also inherited bluntness. "How are you, Grandma?" she asks. "I was hoping to see you looking stronger by now. You look exhausted." "Well, thank you very much. And how have you been, my dear?" the grandmother answers with forced humor. The granddaughter, half-smiling, weighs pressing her grandmother about her health but then simply answers her question. "We've been gener-ally fine," she says. "The children wear me out. But you know I wouldn't have it any other way." As if on cue, the 5-year-old girl runs into the room and pulls at the granddaughter's arm to make her come to the kitchen. The granddaughter gets up, says "I'll be back," and fol-lows her daughter down the hall. The grandmother finds herself alone again, feeling forgotten in the ridiculous room. She wonders if it would be rude to go back up to her bedroom. Just then the granddaughter hur-ries back in without her child and flops onto the floral couch.

"Mom just told me your chemo's done and you're feeling much better," the granddaughter exclaims. The grandmother replies vaguely,

"I'm coming along." The granddaughter frowns and says, "I know my mother believes whatever she wants. But I don't think you look yourself. Tell me what's going on with you." The grandmother looks at her dourly and says, "I'm not really sure what's going on. All I know is that I'm just tired." "The doctors predict you'll bounce back now that the chemo's over," the granddaughter hastens to reassure her. But the grandmother's downcast expression doesn't change. "I don't think I'll be doing much more bouncing," she says. "I'll be lucky if I do much more living. I don't see much chance of ever being myself again. The thought of fighting hard just to linger on exhausts me." The granddaughter is momentarily stunned, then says anxiously, "Mother never told me you felt like this. To me, you're still yourself, just sitting here and talking with me. I don't care if you can't cook the family dinners anymore. I want you here with me, with my kids, so they can get to know you." The grandmother reaches over and touches her hand. "That's very kind of you to say," the old woman says quietly. "I would like to be here with you as long as I can."

The doorbell rings again; more grandchildren and their families have arrived. The 5-year-old girl comes running into the living room again and then veers toward the sound of the boisterous greetings at the front door. "Go ahead," the grandmother says to her favorite granddaughter. "Go to your child. We'll talk after dinner. I'm content to sit here for a while."

In the dining room later, the family matriarch sits stiffly at the head of the long table between her two daughters. A gaggle of husbands, granddaughters, and babbling great-grandchildren sits in closely set folding chairs along either side. The older and younger sisters beam as they watch their own daughters fussing with the fidgety children. The matriarch, tonight's birthday girl, takes only a distracted interest in the excitement at the table's younger end. No one comments about the fact that she barely samples the turkey thigh on her plate; that her carrots and scalloped potatoes haven't been touched goes unnoticed. When, toward the meal's end, the older sister brings out a large, white-frosted sheet cake with pink roses and lettering, the grandmother puts on a wan smile as she feels the whole family's eyes on her. "You shouldn't have gone to this trouble," says the grandmother. "It's your birthday, Mom," answers the younger sister. "You really should not have done this," the grandmother repeats. When the older sister says sweetly, "Why don't you be gracious for a change, Mom?" the smile evaporates from the grandmother's face. The older sister continues in a louder voice, addressing the entire table, "We're here to celebrate you, Mother. You've done so well with your treatments. Everybody, look how well she's done." The grandmother puts the smile back on and says weakly, "Thank you all." She adds to her daughters, "Why don't you cut some good-sized pieces for the children," then leans against the back of her chair, looking drained.

After the children have been shooed from the table, the plates have been stacked and cleared, and the smell of percolating coffee wafts from the kitchen, the grandmother excuses herself to go rest for a little while. Her favorite granddaughter volunteers to help her to her bedroom. As they slowly inch toward the staircase, the older sister calls out to her eldest child, "Hurry back down before your coffee gets cold." But, 15 minutes later, the granddaughter hasn't yet returned. Standing at the bottom of the stairs, the older sister can make out the murmur of their low voices upstairs but not their words. When the granddaughter finally returns to the table 5 minutes later, her jaw is set in anger.

"Is your coffee cold? What took you so long? Do you want a slice of pie?" the older sister asks in quick succession. The granddaughter sits down at her place without looking at her mother. "You know I was talking with Grandma," she says tersely. "Someone has got to take the time to listen to her and not just patronize her." The older sister places her cup down in its saucer and says in a cold voice, "And what is that supposed to mean?" The granddaughter says, "You think just because she finished chemo she's better. But she says she's not better. She feels like hell. But you don't want to see that." The younger sister suddenly blurts out to her sibling, "I've been telling you Mother's still depressed." For a moment, the granddaughter and the older daughter glare at each other, ignoring the younger sister's comment. Then the granddaughter turns toward her aunt and replies angrily. "Yeah, she's depressed. So, what have you and my mother done about it?" The older sister clears her throat and says self-righteously, "I am here with her every day. I have given up my job to be here all day. So, who are you to come traipsing in for the first time in months and inform me what is really going on with my mother? I can see very well what she's like." The granddaughter doesn't back down. "You don't see what she's like," she says. "You're wrong. I do," the older sister insists. "So, why don't you go upstairs and talk with her yourself?" the granddaughter challenges her.

The older sister looks around at her daughter, sister, and the few other adults still picking at their desserts and then pushes herself away from the table. She clambers upstairs, knocks on her mother's bedroom door, and then lets herself in without waiting for her mother's reply. "I hear you've been complaining about me to your favorite granddaughter," she declares while standing in the doorway. "That's not true," the mother answers calmly while lying on her bed with a crocheted blanket thrown over her legs. "What is the matter?" "What did you say to her?" the older sister demands. "I told her I feel very tired, and I have a sinking feeling about how this is all going to turn out," the mother responds. "If your daughter thinks you haven't gotten that, then she reached that conclusion on her own." The older sister pauses to regain her composure, then says with less anger, "I thought you were doing better." The mother replies, "I am very grateful the chemo is over. But I feel plain lousy all the time. I can't help feeling that way for now." The older sister responds defensively, "I've tried very hard to take good care of you." "I know you have," answers the mother, "and my not feeling well or hopeful is not a criticism of anything you've done for me. Don't take it personally." The older sister glances at the floor and then looks up at her mother again. "We can talk more about all this after everyone leaves, I suppose," she says a little reluctantly. "Yes, I'd like that," replies the mother. "Go back down to your guests. I'll be down in a little while." When the older sister turns toward the door to leave, she wears a lined face of frustration.

After years and decades of living together, you thoroughly know your loved one's personality, tendencies, and outlooks. After weeks and months of providing care to him, you know firsthand how those attributes are affected by illness's symptoms, prognoses, and treatments. But being so close to your sick relative can sometimes create a kind of myopia. Your lifelong knowledge of him can distort, not enhance, your understanding of how he's now feeling and functioning. Your day-to-day attentiveness to his needs can skew your perception of his desires. As paradoxical as it sounds, when you're intimately familiar with the person you're caring for, you may lose, or never gain, full awareness of the awfulness of what is happening to him.

This is not altogether bad. Chapters 2 and 5 explored some of the defenses people employ to avoid being overwhelmed by the uncertainties of a serious illness. Denial and minimization may have helped you take on caregiving when the crisis occurred by allowing you to downplay the enormity of the task. With the same sleight of hand you may now maintain your ability to hope and persevere through the course of the illness.

Awareness can also be worn down by the rough daily grind. Early on in a medical crisis, you hover by your ill loved one's bed full of concern, wincing at every groan, running yourself ragged to meet every need. But as time passes and the crisis settles into a prolonged chronic phase, your days are less fueled by anxiety than guided by routine. Faced with a loved one who can no longer dress and feed herself, you're initially shocked by having to dress and feed her yourself, then master the skills involved, and then, after many repetitions, approach the tasks with the same half-conscious competence that you would any other chores. Faced with a demented relative who can no longer take his own pills, you're confused by the tablets' many shapes and colors until experience makes you an expert on their administration and side effects. The new skills you dutifully practice usually become second nature within a matter of weeks. For many of you, they seem to become first nature. Family caregiver becomes your primary identity. The schedule of daily caregiving chores, weekly medical appointments, and monthly prescription refills, like the sun's rising or the moon's phases, comes to set the rhythm and structure of your life.

There are clear advantages to giving your life over to a caregiving routine in this way. Foremost among them is that you no longer have to think very much about some of the unpleasant things you must do but instead can fulfill your duties while coasting on automatic pilot. Disengaging your mind to a degree usually cuts down on the feeling of drudgery. It also distances you emotionally each time you have to bathe or toilet a previously dignified and independent loved one.

The trouble is that the same disengagement is also a disadvantage. It may mean your awareness of your loved one's plight and the gradual changes brought on by a slowly progressing disease, for instance, is no longer so acute. The days blur together; changes pass unnoticed; the humdrum of caregiving is taken for granted. It can also mean you lose emotional attunement with your loved one himself. You hear the groans of his suffering, but they no longer provoke a visceral reaction in you. You see him struggling, but you now respond first by thinking about what you have to do for him rather than empathizing with the humiliation he may be feeling. It's not that, under the yoke of routine, you care less than you once did at the beginning of the medical crisis. It's that your immersion in routines places blinders on you that focus your attention on the day's tasks and can obscure your view of the disease's arc or the ill person's diminishment.

This sounds cold and perhaps implausible. Family caregiving is, above all else, a loving endeavor. Why would you commit to helping a loved one and then distance yourself emotionally from that person? The answer is that this isn't a conscious decision but a side effect of a state of prolonged, unremitting duress. You develop a callus at a spot of continual pressure. You become, if not callous, then numb when continuously strained by caregiving rigors and the spectacle of your loved one's decline. Becoming gradually less attuned to the suffering around you (let alone your own suffering) is a way of surviving emotionally to keep on doing what needs to be done. A natural outgrowth of this is that you settle into rigid routines of care, going through the daily motions of tending and feeding like a mindless creature of habit. Losing awareness and flexibility in these ways does protect you by helping you feel and think less. But it has corrosive effects as well.

Take, for example, the older sister. As long as she's carting laundry, slamming cupboards, and scrubbing dishes, she's not pacing the kitchen and wringing her hands over cancer's threat. It's not that she doesn't think about what might happen. But these concerns are pushed aside just enough so they don't occupy all her waking thoughts. Instead, she's maintaining what sense of control over the household routine she can manage during an inherently uncontrollable medical crisis; it undoubtedly helps her cope. In the process, however, two changes take place. First, a certain distancing occurs from the mother's condition and Mother herself. Not only does Mom stop feeling heard when her daughter is rushing about, but she begins to feel like a burden—another onerous chore to be checked off some list. Second, the daughter comes to follow her routines habitually and inflexibly to ensure her sense of control even if they're no longer the best strategies for helping Mom. These changes can only add to the feelings of worthlessness that have plagued the mother since she developed cancer. They can only deepen her depression.

Or imagine the middle-aged wife of an elderly man who has suffered several strokes. She amazes herself with all she handles deftly—cooking and spoon-feeding him three pureed meals a day; dressing, undressing, and sponge-bathing him daily; even hoisting him on her back to and from the toilet. But while she goes to bed each night satisfied with her accomplishments, she also dreads tomorrow's heavy chores. Somewhere along the line, several transformations occur. The man who was once her beloved spouse is now mostly a challenging patient. She stops interacting with him emotionally as her life partner and more as the inanimate object of her herculean efforts. She pursues those efforts each day in a rigid, unthinking manner to protect herself from becoming upset. If the physical wear and tear of caregiving takes a toll on her body, these shifts in perspective sap her energy and spirit. Gone is the revivifying effect of feeling she's in a mutual loving relationship. Gone, too, is the capacity to flexibly solve new problems as conditions evolve. Completing chores gives her little more than the assurance she has held on for another day. This may lead her to conclude she's been victimized by his strokes. This can only increase the likelihood she'll one day burn out.

Are you losing awareness of yourself and your ill loved one?
- Do you find yourself denying changes that others point out to you?
- Do you really look at your ill loved one or see her only with your mind's eye, as she used to be?
- When your relative calls out to you, do you automatically shift into problem-solving mode to prevent yourself from reacting with anger or frustration or resentment?
- Do you take refuge in routine?

It may seem counterintuitive that the key to preventing burnout or keeping a sick relative from feeling like a burden is to increase, not decrease, your awareness of all aspects of the medical and family predicaments and to greet each day with a fresh outlook, open to change. Increasing awareness means facing down the terrors of illness to remain connected with your loved one. It means avoiding being lulled into numbness and adopting inflexible routines. The trouble with all this, of course, is that limiting awareness of what you're feeling and simply following set routines have been unconscious means of protecting yourself from being emotionally overwhelmed. How can you heighten your awareness of your failing loved one without amplifying your worst fears? How can you flexibly modify what you do without feeding your anxiety?

In the past 15 years, the term "mindfulness" has entered the mainstream of American psychology and healthcare, spawning scores of pop psych books and instructional videos and launching dozens of community programs. The word is meant to capture the idea that, by directing where you focus your attention, you can shape your reactions to life's problems.

The mindfulness movement has been spurred by Buddhist thinker Thich Nhat Hanh and former University of Massachusetts professor Jon Kabat-Zinn, who have sought to employ Eastern meditative practices to assuage Western turmoil and stress. "Mindfulness," writes Dr. Kabat-Zinn in his 1990 book *Full Catastrophe Living*, is "remembering to be present in all our waking moments. . . . We learn to be aware of our fears and our pain, yet at the same time . . . empowered by a connection to something deeper within ourselves, a discerning wisdom that helps to penetrate and transcend the fear and the pain, and to discover some peace and hope within our situation *as it is* [his emphasis]." It's not resignation or even necessarily acceptance of a terrible situation; practicing mindfulness is emphatically not a form of giving up. It's a kind of surrendering, however—to the power derived from facing reality with eyes open and senses sharpened so as to take in every nuance and wrinkle, even every noxious event. Mindfulness is also not an escape into some mental la-la land or a deadening of feelings. It's an enhanced awareness of the here and now in which your emotions may well up in response but never drown out your connection with the surrounding world. And it doesn't thwart daily care routines, only the mindlessness bred by rote inflexibility.

There's a general methodology for learning to be more aware while increasing your sense of what Kabat-Zinn called "peace and hope." He and others recommend a host of techniques for heightening attention while also stilling the mind's knee-jerk emotional reactions—reactions that can make it more difficult to respond to circumstances appropriately and effectively. Chief among the techniques is the Eastern practice of meditation—sitting motionlessly, breathing evenly and deeply, and focusing your thoughts on a phrase, sound, or image. At first glance it seems simple: What could be easier than sitting and breathing? But it's the third component that can be maddeningly elusive. The mind's thoughts are like mercury. Instead of resting on one topic, they have a tendency to slip and slither in all directions, scattering the bright beads of your awareness. Through the regular practice of sitting, breathing, and focusing, you can learn to contain your thoughts and settle your mind. Then you can calmly maintain your awareness of present circumstances, fully taking in the richness of every moment, and be prepared to change flexibly as those circumstances warrant. Considerations of the past and future aren't excluded from mindful meditation.

Rather, you remain cognizant of how past events have brought you to the present juncture without ruminating distractedly about what has already happened. Or you ponder possible paths ahead without being wracked by worries about the future.

Most family caregivers are already too hard-pressed for time and money even to consider taking intensive courses in meditation. (In an ideal world, such training would help all of us handle everyday stressors and crises with greater poise and equanimity.) Fortunately, elements of mindfulness can be fostered in other ways to allow you to remain attuned to your ill loved one and open to new ways of caregiving without overtaxing your psyche.

To mention one simple example, keeping a diary or journal of your experiences from the beginning of a medical crisis to its conclusion allows you to meet mindfulness' two requirements. It sharpens awareness by helping you step out of the onrush of medical events and the drudgery of daily care to notice more carefully how your loved one is changing and how you are being affected by caregiving. Even when you engage in merely descriptive writing—for example, lists of chores or observations of how well a loved one eats or sleeps—you're reflecting on the caregiving to which you're committed rather than simply being caught up in its vortex of reflexive day-to-day existing. Because diary entries can be reread at a later date, they also promote an awareness of the continuity of the family's experience as members persevere through the different phases of the illness. At the same time, keeping diaries can be soothing. Some people consider the process of writing itself to be a quasi-meditative act. It requires an absorbed concentration, an inner clarifying of feelings and thoughts, and a weighing and measuring of words that can induce a creative reverie. The practiced writer emerges from the writing session with mind focused and calmed.

Other means are available for you to promote increased awareness or calmness or both. By participating in caregiver or disease-specific support groups, online discussion groups, or web blogs, you can learn about others' experiences and consequently gain a basis for comparing and contrasting your own. More important, you're generally called on in these groups to tell the stories of how you're being affected by the missions you've undertaken. Just grappling with your complex experience to the degree that you can put it into words fosters reflection. When those words then elicit questions or emotional responses from group members, you experience your own story differently. That frequently alters how you see yourself and allows you to approach giving care in more flexible, imaginative ways.

Then there are activities you can take on by yourself without the support of others. Many bookstores and websites sell relaxation tapes or CDs (such as those by Kabat-Zinn) that instruct the listener in the kinds of deep-breathing exercises and directed visualization techniques that psychologists frequently teach those with anxiety or chronic pain. They're intended to bring about a state of increased calm so the listener can more effectively face life's stressors. Yoga offers similar benefits. While many people think of it primarily as a means of stretching and relaxing the body, it's also a way of stilling and relaxing the mind. Finally—and perhaps most profoundly— prayer works wonders by increasing awareness and inducing calm. By appealing to a higher power, you mentally remove yourself from the mire of daily routines and perceive your struggles within the bigger picture of a universal plan or ultimate authority. The act of praying—often involving quiet contemplation, slow, rhythmic breathing, and the repetition of well-worn phrases or chants—can elicit a relaxed state similar to that meditation promises. (For more on the topic of spirituality, see Chapter 8.)

Ways to foster awareness:
- Keep a diary or journal.
- Talk—and listen—to members of a support group.
- Go online—vent, query, share, commiserate.
- Learn mindfulness, relaxation, and visualization techniques from a CD/tape or book—public libraries are full of them.
- Take a yoga class.
- Pray.

Regardless of your method, increasing awareness brings several rewards. If you can remain cognizant of the progression of your loved one's plight without becoming overwhelmed, you no longer need to stay locked into rigid routines of daily chores to steady yourself. You can listen more carefully to your loved one's concerns and then respond to them in a more attuned fashion. This will mean soberly noting and considering each change in the patient and then flexibly tweaking your caregiving to suit developing conditions and needs. You'll be a better problem solver because your thinking won't be confined to the limits of the routines you've established; instead, you'll have the latitude to be more innovative. In general, greater awareness and flexibility will also mean gaining a clearer view of the whole medical situation, thereby leading you to strike the right balance of hope and acceptance. That will make you more resilient throughout the medical crisis.

Developing awareness helps you:
- Hear what your loved one really needs.
- Stay connected to the real person before you rather than clinging to an image from the past.
- Achieve cautious optimism.
- Respond to your relative as a person you love rather than as a "to do" list.
- Accept and learn from your emotional responses instead of distracting yourself with tasks to accomplish—the best way to avoid burnout.

At mid-morning Saturday on the day after the party, the older sister wakes up later than usual and finds her husband's side of the bed is already cold. Though she can hear the clatter of breakfast under way downstairs, she continues to lie in bed, feeling stiff-limbed and grumpy. She spent half the night stewing about last evening's events and now takes up some of the same thoughts again. Part of her feels humiliated. Her daughter showed her up with her mother—in front of the rest of the family, no less. For that she could crown her. But another part of her is angry that her mother sided with her daughter. And then, to top it off, the two of them appeared to be in cahoots against her. This is her measure of thanks, she broods, for giving up large parts of her life over the years to help each of them. Wrapping herself in the blankets, she drifts into darker thoughts. Well, when the cancer takes Mother, I won't have to deal with this much longer, she says to herself. Then, almost immediately, she pushes that thought away, telling herself firmly that Mother is going to be fine. Discomfited by the direction her mind is taking, she arises suddenly, puts on her robe and slippers, and scurries downstairs.

She's apprehensive about seeing her mother this morning. She wonders if Mom will give her a chiding look when she walks into the kitchen, as if to say "We still need to have our little talk." Or will Mother simply give her a scolding look for sleeping so late and not preparing her breakfast? The older sister is also anxious about the kitchen itself. She never finished washing all the pots and pans in the sink last night before she collapsed from fatigue, and now her husband has likely added more layers of greasy utensils. But as the older sister enters the room and glances at the sink, she's surprised to see it's been emptied and scoured. She looks over to the kitchen table and observes her husband and mother picking at the last scraps of their cheese omelets. Sitting next to them pouring juice, she's shocked to see, is her eldest daughter.

"What's wrong? Something's happened. Where are the kids?" the older sister asks shrilly.

"The kids are home," the daughter responds. "Nothing's wrong. Why don't you sit down and have some of the omelet I made?"

The older sister's husband jumps up from his chair to make room for his wife. "Here, honey, sit down," he says. "I have things to do." He dumps his plate and cup in the sink and, without making eye contact, hurries past her to go down to the basement.

The older sister now looks at her daughter and mother suspiciously. Something must be up. She sits down, pours herself some coffee, and waits. There's an awkward silence. Then Mother says, "I'm tired. Why don't I head back upstairs and let the two of you talk?" "I'll help you back upstairs, Grandma," says the daughter. "No," says the older sister firmly. "I will."

The older sister comes back downstairs, takes her seat, and waits again. The daughter pushes a piece of toast around her plate and then looks up and says, "I couldn't sleep last night. I felt terrible about how I behaved toward you. I came over to talk about it."

The older sister, still wary, leans forward in her chair. She says, "Considering what happened, I didn't get much sleep either," then waits for her daughter to go on and explain herself. The daughter puts the toast down and says, "I know how you are. I know how hard this has been for you. Dad probably hasn't been much help. I should have been a little easier on you."

"How would you know how hard this has been for me?" the older sister asks brusquely. The daughter ignores the anger in her mother's tone and continues in a conciliatory way, saying, "When things get tough, you're always the one to put your nose to the grindstone. I re-member how you kept everyone going when your father was sick. I see you doing the same with Grandma. You take care of everything. But you're so intent on keeping things on track that I think you overlook some things. The emotional stuff, I mean."

"Don't try to imply I'm not having feelings about what's going on with your grandmother," the older sister retorts. "Nobody is feeling more about her than I am. Not you, for instance." The daughter is quiet for a moment. She then says sadly, "I don't want to fight with you. That's the opposite of why I'm here this morning. I'm worried about you just as I'm worried about Grandma. There's such a thing as being too efficient in doing everything that has to be done. I know; I'm just like you. I get so wrapped up in completing the thousand daily things with the kids that I don't pay attention to how they're feeling a lot of the time—or how I'm feeling either."

The older sister is silently thoughtful. She regards her daughter and sees she's in earnest. "I'm not entirely sure what you're saying," she says, forcing herself to speak in a milder tone. "What is it you want me to do?"

"It's too easy to get caught up in all the things we have to do," the daughter says. "We have to help each other stay in close touch with Grandma—knowing what she's feeling physically and emotionally so we can change what we're doing to help her as well as we can. We don't know how much longer we're going to have her."

The older sister is beginning to feel patronized again. "And how are we supposed to do this?" she asks, an irritable note creeping back into her voice.

The daughter hears her mother's irritation and continues more sheepishly. "I'm not exactly sure," she says. "I think Grandma probably has told me things she won't tell you because she's afraid of hurting you. She says you take everything too personally." The older sister's eyes widen momentarily. The daughter goes on, "I don't have to be here under your feet all the time. You know I can't anyway because I have to take care of my kids. Perhaps if we e-mailed back and forth about our impressions of what's happening to Grandma and how we're thinking and feeling about it, we could stay in touch better and be more aware of everything that's going on. It's an idea I read about on a health website. Because I can't be around very much, it would give me a chance to put my two cents in; you know I need to do that. But I could also point out things to help you that you may not be seeing because you're so close to the situation. It could be like our own support group."

The older sister, face expressionless, says nothing. Her daughter, thinking that her mother is offended by the idea, says quickly, "I'm not saying I think you need a lot of support. I'm just saying we could keep ourselves more in touch with what's happening medically and emotionally so we all could cope better." The older sister says in a low voice, almost begrudgingly, "I think it's a good idea." The daughter responds with surprise: "You do?" Then, realizing her mother is serious, she grows more enthusiastic. "We could put your sister on the e-mail list," she says. "And my sisters, too. It would be good for us all to write to each other. Writing helps me think things through and calm down. I think we'll fight less if we're all writing regularly. And Grandma will feel we're really with her as she goes through this."

The daughter looks pleased with herself. The older sister waits patiently for her to finish, then says: "Okay, I'm willing to try it your way. When Grandma first got sick, I used to write in a little journal late at night about what was going on, but I've just been so busy lately. I agree writing makes things clearer. I think reading about how you and the others see things will keep me from focusing only on what needs to get done every day and maybe help me think about doing things differently."

"Good," says the daughter. "That's the idea."

"But," the older sister enunciates, "this e-mailing isn't going to make me any calmer if you and your sisters use it to criticize me. I don't need you to tell me what I should do. This isn't a democracy. I have to make the decisions about what Grandma needs. If you want to make me more aware of things, that's fine, but no pot shots."

"I'm not going to do that," says the daughter defensively. "That's not the point."

"And, by the way," the older sister continues, "I'm tired of doing almost everything for Grandma myself. Do you think I can use this e-mail support group to ask you and your sisters for some specific help sometimes? Or is it only for the purpose of making us more aware and calmer?"

The daughter sighs. "You can ask away. When I can, I'll come," she says. Thinking her mother is finished, she gets up to take her plate to the sink when her mother touches her firmly on the arm to make her sit back down.

"Just one more thing," says the older sister, "but it's the most important thing. You love your grandmother very much. But you won't know it's not the same as having a mother with deadly sickness until you have to take care of me one day. There are days I feel so terrible about my mother having cancer that I don't want to be more aware of it. There are times when there's no possible way I'm going to be calmer. I have to shield myself sometimes. I'm going to."

The daughter sits there quietly, looking at her mother with sympathy. "Maybe you're right that I can't understand the way you feel entirely," she says. "All the more reason we should write to each other. I do want to understand you better. I really don't want to give you a hard time."

"Okay, then," says the older sister curtly, jumping up and taking the daughter's plate and cup to the sink herself.

Fostering awareness and flexibility is the best way for families to prepare themselves to adjust to the many changing conditions brought on by a long-lasting serious illness. One of the most deleterious potential changes is the neglect of other family needs as a loved one's health wanes and caregiving of him consumes greater family resources. Family members need to learn to conserve themselves and to consider their own requirements for caring. Patients need to find ways of giving back love for the care they are receiving. In the next chapter, we will explore ways of preserving all family relationships during a prolonged medical crisis, but especially protecting intimacy.

A Mother Changed by Stroke

Q: *As an only child, I feel solely responsible for the well-being of my elderly mother. During most of my life, we've had a wonderful relationship. But after relocating 2½ years ago to her house to take care of her after she had a serious stroke, I find myself unable to deal with her. I can't stand her constant criticism and moping about. She doesn't have a word of thanks for me and seems oblivious to the fact I've given up my own life. Whenever she gives me her look of exasperation, I feel like screaming at her. She's changed or I have, but we're not working together well. This has become a nightmare.*

A: It's terribly distressing to devote yourself to caring for a parent only to have your relationship with her suffer as a result. You need to reflect on and address three factors to remedy this predicament: the ways your mother has changed, the alterations in your reactions to her, and the negative cycle that has come to dominate the interactions between the two of you.

First, let's consider your mother. Stroke, like traumatic brain injury, brain cancer, and other brain insults, often changes people's moods and personalities. There's a strong likelihood the changes you perceive in your mom are due to neurological damage she's experienced. In addition, having to depend on you for care may be depressing her. Both factors may prevent her from being the person with whom you had so wonderful a relationship. I'd recommend talking with her physician about possibly treating her depression and thereby modifying her sour behavior to some extent. Even more important, though, is for you to modify your expectations of her.

Are you aware that you expect your mother to act as she always did? If not, then I'd suggest stepping back and reflecting some more. It's extremely difficult to accept that a loved one has been altered to the point of unfamiliarity. If you know you expect your mother to be her old self, you may need to grieve the loss of the person you've known. That's an essential step toward figuring out how to get along with who she's become. It's understandable that the ungratefulness and moodiness you see make you want to scream. Instead, try the following:

• Remember she's been changed by her stroke. You don't have to excuse bad behavior, but you must take into account that it may have a neurological basis that's not your mother's fault. By viewing her behavior as a symptom and not a personal affront, you will decrease the intensity of your reaction. Talk with her physician about how you think your mother has changed and learn what's reasonable to expect from her.

• When riled, leave the room or house to get greater distance from her and your emotions. You'll have more control over your reactions if you have the time and space to think them through. You can also use mindfulness, deep breathing, or relaxation techniques to stay aware of your feelings without feeding anger or letting it fester.

• Arrange for respite care through other relatives and friends so you aren't on duty all the time.

• If it's still so painful to deal with the changes she's undergone that you have one hand permanently clamped over your mouth, consider getting treatment (psychotherapeutic and/or pharmacologic) for yourself to mitigate your own likely burnout and depression.

• Finally, it's vital to gain greater awareness of the interactions between the two of you. I'd venture to guess that the more your mom mopes, the more disconcerted you get. The more disconcerted you get, the more she feels resented and then mopes. You can break this cycle by intentionally reacting to her depressed or critical behavior with extra dollops of understanding and kindness. That may not induce her to be who she was, but will stop the escalating antagonism between the two of you and give you half a chance to learn to appreciate who she is.

Planning for Caregiver Illness

Q: *One night recently I came down with a high fever and really felt like I couldn't move. By the next day I had a terrible sore throat too. Fortunately, my niece was able to come over and take care of Mom for a few hours while I went to the doctor, but then it turned out I had strep throat and really shouldn't be exposing my mother to the infection, especially in her weakened condition. I had to leave Mom without a lot of her needs met until my niece could come over again after work. But I can't count on her being available like that, especially with no notice. What are family caregivers supposed to do when we get sick?*

A: Who but an around-the-clock caregiver can better attest to the saying "There's no rest for the weary"? And yet your question is proof that proper rest is essential, because no caregiver, however superhuman, is immune from fatigue and sickness. Putting together an emergency "when-I-get-sick" plan, ideally with a decision tree of options to address an array of foreseeable contingencies, is essential.

The first step in such planning isn't usually identifying resources, though, but mustering willingness. Three factors frequently get in the way: guilt, magical thinking, and one-day-at-a-time coping. Some caregivers are so convinced it's their ill loved ones and not themselves who deserve care that even planning for emergency self-care is guilt-provoking for them. Others hold superstitious ideas that planning for maladies is tantamount to inviting fate to inflict them on the family. Many are so focused on getting through their daily rigors hour by hour that they haven't the inclination or foresight to plan for tomorrow's possible hardships. As common as these attitudes may be, they are neither logical nor helpful. The caregiver who's too inflexible to prepare for sickness or other misfortunes is at risk for letting down her loved one when they eventually occur.

So, what aid is needed in an emergency? The answer in your case was someone to come to your home, provide company and supervision for your mom, and even help her hands-on with lifting and dressing. A simple get-well card, while thoughtful, was not going to cut it. Caregivers generally look to family, community, and professional resources to meet those sorts of practical needs.

Your niece's proximity and willingness were revealed for the blessing that they are. Family is often the prime resource in an emergency. Rather than waiting for crunch time to plead with an adult child, sibling, or other relative to step up and help, it's better to ask that person when all is well what he or she is willing and capable of doing in the event you are indisposed. Verbal commitments in advance aren't guarantees of timely action but increase the likelihood a family member will come through if and when the need arises.

Unfortunately, many caregivers don't have interested relatives available or in close proximity. Canvassing resources in your local community would be a next step. Good, generous, and able-bodied neighbors to help dress your mother, pick up groceries, or drop off casseroles are indispensable in the short term. For those involved with a church, synagogue, or mosque, many religious institutions have volunteer committees to visit the ill, provide driving to and from doctors' offices, and do simple household chores.

Professional resources should also be tapped. The key questions for your loved one's physician (or yours) or a social worker regard the availability of respite and home healthcare services. Many counties (generally through their Area Agencies on Aging) will have information on means for the caregivers of elderly citizens to get urgent, intensive assistance. Some insurance companies have provisions for placement of the patient in a skilled nursing facility on a temporary basis while the caregiver is incapacitated.

Of course, lining up all of these resources, as well as any others available to you, is better than planning to rely on just one. And learning now about who to contact and what they can offer will reduce your reticence about calling for help when an emergency strikes. There's no formula for warding off sickness, only best-laid plans to maximize the well-being of both your loved one and yourself under any conditions.

When Dad Resists Assisted Living

Q: *My 85-year-old father has been diagnosed with the early stages of dementia. He still lives alone and drives, though only in his own small neighborhood, to the grocery store and post office and the like. He's been told by his doctor he has dementia and that it's okay to live alone and drive in his limited capacity. My sister and I wish he'd move into an assisted living facility, but he adamantly refuses. What can we do?*

A: This is an excruciating predicament faced by thousands of American families each year. It pits the desire to allow a failing elder to maintain control over his life against the fervent wish to keep that loved one safe (not to mention protecting any pedestrians and other drivers who may cross his path). There are two possible tacks for you to take; both require subtle persuasion.

The first tack involves the manner in which you and your sister approach your father. His degree of dementia is unclear from your description. Assuming that he's still capable of reasoning, I'd suggest appealing to his capacity to choose wisely rather than trying to overpower him by the force of your combined pressure. In other words, express your concerns for his safety, ask him to indulge you by visiting an assisted living facility with you, but don't challenge his right to decide for himself whether he wants to live there. Most of us are more likely to change our position and lifestyle if such a transformation is of our own choosing; placed under duress to change, we typically resist, regardless of the soundness of the other person's arguments.

If your father isn't capable of thinking through the consequences of his choices, then you may have to take the tack of relying on his physician to facilitate change. I'd make an appointment with his doctor to provide information and express your concerns about how he's managing day to day. Tell the physician explicitly you don't believe your father is safe living alone or driving even locally (especially if he's being prescribed a sedating Alzheimer's drug such as Aricept or Exelon). Physicians are generally cautious by nature or for fear of malpractice suits. While he or she may disagree with your assessment, the doctor is unlikely to be so cavalier as to completely dismiss your perspective. If you ask him or her to require your father to undergo the kind of extensive driving evaluations for older adults available at most physical medicine rehabilitation hospitals, the physician will probably comply. Should Father fail that evaluation, the physician will notify his state's department of motor vehicles not to renew his license. (Most states have laws that mandate doctors to report impaired drivers.) Should he pass the driver's evaluation, then you can feel greater assurance he is in fact safe to drive in his neighborhood.

Here's one more strategy. Since most dementias are progressive, it's likely your father's condition will get worse. If his physician still contends that Father is now capable of living independently, ask him or her when he'll probably need greater help. At the least, you can establish a possible timeline and functional parameters that will clue in everybody involved, including Dad, when it'll finally be time for him to sell the house and car and accept assistance.

A Mother in Decline, a Father in Denial

Q: *For the past 15 years, my father has been taking care of my mother, who has the progressing–remitting type of multiple sclerosis. Recently my two siblings and I have been worried he's so set in his ways that he isn't taking into account that she continues to go downhill. He still insists on doing everything for her, despite the fact that we're always volunteering to help the two of them. He even argues with us that her condition is stable and that she hasn't gotten worse in a long time. We love him and don't want to see him wear himself out because he won't open his eyes and change his caregiving ways. What should we do?*

A: Your father is doing yeoman's work with diligence and pride. Hopefully, you and your siblings are frequently praising his efforts. You're also right, though, to be concerned about his well-being. Raising his awareness of your mother's condition is probably the best way to help him not be so rigid about his caregiving routines. But I can almost guarantee he won't be enthused about having his awareness raised; I'm sure he prefers seeing his wife as stable and resists other perceptions. If he's stubbornly wrong, however, he may be setting himself up to burn out. That could only negatively impact your mom.

If you try to share your own perception of how Mom is declining, he may dismiss what you say out of hand because you're his child (regardless of being an adult) or because he feels you don't see your mother often enough to be an accurate judge. You'll likely have to bring in your mother's healthcare team to make him reconsider his views. I'd suggest calling her neurologist about holding a family meeting to discuss where she is in her disease process and what the prognosis is for the decline in her functioning. If your mother has also seen a physiatrist (physical medicine rehab doctor) or physical therapist lately, it would be helpful for him or her to join the meeting as well. Please ask the professionals to bring whatever quantifiable data they have on your mom—for instance, Mini-Mental Status Exam scores or FIM (Functional Independence Measure) scores, commonly used in rehab. Then invite your dad to the meeting. He may be angry that you requested it without conferring with him first, but I doubt he'll miss it. (Depending on your mother's condition, you may want her to be present, too, or just summarize the information for her later.) Your father may discount the professionals' observations but will have trouble ignoring numerical data that suggest your mother's decline is proceeding through periodic exacerbations. They'll also present potential scenarios for the kind of help she's likely to need in the future.

The idea isn't to overwhelm your father with incontrovertible evidence that your mother is getting worse, but rather to broaden his awareness of what's occurring, to assist him in preparing to take care of your mother as well as possible. With that new information and whatever recommendations the professionals make for caring for your mom, you and your siblings will be in a better position to persuade your dad to accept more of your help. But you mustn't say "I told you so" to him. Be respectful of his pride as a devoted husband and caregiver. Instead, gently extend your offer again to pitch in. If he regards you as sincere, supportive, and caring, there's a chance he'll take it.

Progressive Illness Changes a Marriage

Q: *I don't like how my father's providing care to my mother has changed their relationship. They had always set an example of the perfect marriage for all of us kids—you know, the kind of couple who never seems to fall out of love or take each other for granted. You'd think that, because my dad is now staying home with my mother more, they'd be even closer. But sometimes I sense my dad being a little more distant from Mom when I'm over there and he's doing all the usual things for her. I know he still loves her very much, and this breaks my heart. What can I do to help?*

A: A good friend of mine was concerned that looking after her mother—a frail older woman who moved into an assisted living facility near her—would eventually feel like a chore and cause her to become emotionally distant from her mom. She came up with a great idea to help avoid this. While on most days she runs errands for her mother or chauffeurs her around, one evening a week she and her husband go to the mother's assisted living facility for the sheer pleasure of dining together. It's a way for them to remember what they value in each other by separating what they have to do for her from what they enjoy doing with her. It's prevented their relationships from being completely defined by care-giving's many duties.

A relationship between a husband and wife is of greater intimacy than that between a daughter and mother, and living together is more challenging than living nearby. But there are still lessons from my friend's situation that can be applied to your parents'. The first is for them to make as sharp a demarcation as possible between time devoted to their caregiving relationship and that devoted to their spousal relationship. The second is to increase their closeness by enhancing their relationship's mutuality.

Both principles demand a heightened awareness on their part of what's going on between your parents at any given moment. Can they intentionally carve out regular time to be together that will not involve caretaking—for example, dinners, movies, necking sessions? It'll require an effort from your dad not to be thinking about what he has to do but to just be with your mom. It'll also necessitate shifting his perspective on her from the focus of his daily work to the source of love in his life. Can she take on a nurturing and giving role toward your dad, or must she always be the recipient of care? If she can take care of your father in some respect—for example, listening to his troubles, rubbing his back—she can engage him as a wife rather than as a patient, and draw your dad closer to her.

If your father drifts along providing care to your mother without an awareness of how doing so affects their relationship, I expect he'll become increasingly distant from your mom. It's better for them to consciously plan changes in their interactions to keep the marital sacrament from deteriorating into wearying and numbing duty.

So, what can you do to help them achieve all this? You can gently suggest that they spend some quality time together and help make it happen by offering to hold down the fort, taking care of some practical chore that will free up some of your dad's time. You might buy them tickets to a play and offer to drop them off and pick them up so they don't have to hassle with transportation. You could bring over a gourmet meal, set the table for them, light the candles, and leave. Then come back and perform some of the nonromantic care functions for your mother that your father usually handles so that the tone of the evening doesn't shift back to caregiving too quickly. If you have siblings, talk to them about how you can all cooperate in this important endeavor.

Of course you may not feel comfortable speaking directly and candidly to either of your parents about this, in which case you should consider whether a trusted peer could broach the subject—a member of the clergy or counselor or even a new therapist or your parents' physician are good possibilities to consider.

CHAPTER SEVEN

Protecting Intimacy

On the morning the mother and the two sisters are scheduled to go over Mother's recent full-body CT scans with the oncologist, they're surprised when the older sister's husband volunteers at breakfast to take time off from work to drive them. Several of the sisters' daughters recently had been pitching in to help—running to the bank, bringing over pans of lasagna—thanks to the older sister's direct pleas on the family's new e-mail support group. But the husband had continued to keep to himself. So, when he made his offer this morning, the older sister looked at him oddly but quickly said yes.

It wasn't that her husband had an especially bad history with the mother; it just wasn't very good either. The two had clashed numerous times long ago when the older sister first began dating him because Mother thought he wasn't bright or educated enough for her daughter. Later there had been some volatile arguments between the husband and mother over Mother's insistence that the older sister's girls be raised with the strictest discipline. After that, Mother and the husband had backed off from each other to a more bearable distance. They weren't exactly indifferent to each other but tended to avoid each other whenever possible. The mother's lengthening convalescence in his home had certainly strained this arrangement. The younger sister's husband had had his clashes, too, with the mother over the years, as well as one memorable explosion with the father about not wanting to attend the funeral of a longtime family friend. But he'd managed in the past decade to become closer to his wife's mother. They had a warmer, teasing rapport than existed between the older sister's standoffish husband and his critical mother-in-law.

Given the past, the older sister is astonished while observing her husband tenderly ushering Mother into the front seat of his SUV and then proceeding to make jokes and encouraging comments to her throughout the short trip to the hospital. "Mom, I'm sure you're going to be all right," he says several times. "These tests are just a formality." Mother, for her part, seems immune to the encouragement or evident change in her son-in-law's behavior and continues looking straight ahead out the window in silence. Sitting in the back, the two sisters glance at each other as if to say, What's up with him?

The husband's sudden concern is not as out of character as it seems. He tends to play hunches, and he's been having a strong one the past few days about this doctor's visit. For weeks he's noticed his mother-in-law dragging around. She's too tough an old bird, he figures, to simply be depressed; he's afraid that, even after extensive surgery and chemo, her cancer has spread. As much as he worries about how his mother-in-law would take such news, he's more concerned about his wife. She's been overstressed for months, alternately hunkered down and frantic. He realizes this is just her way of dealing with an acute crisis. But he misses the easier manner she usually has. Nowadays she collapses into bed late and forces herself out early. They've had few dinners together and no movies or evening talks over tea. What's more, sex has ceased. All of it—not just the lack of sex—has been bothering him for a while, though he hasn't dared to say anything for fear of making her feel worse or becoming the target of her frustrations. But given what he's afraid is coming today, he's decided he should be close at hand to try to help her.

"Why don't you just drop us off by the entrance and then pick us up later?" the older sister tells him as he pulls in front of the hospital. "No, I'd like to come up and join you," he responds before turning into the garage. Mother's face remains impassive, staring straight ahead. The sisters glance at each other again. As he helps his mother-in-law out of the front seat after parking the car, he gives the back of her hand an uncharacteristic pat, which she receives stiffly.

The oncologist keeps them waiting for 40 minutes. The husband chatters amiably about his work and the grandkids to his wife and her sister, although they barely answer back. Finally, the oncologist leads them into his private office, now crammed with an additional chair for the husband. The oncologist makes little small talk but instead gets right down to business. "As you know," he says, directing his comments to the mother, "we sent you for a series of CT scans to assess the state of your recovery after abdominal surgery and to rule out the spread of the cancer to other parts of your body. We used an extended course of chemotherapy to minimize the chances of such spreading from occurring." He pauses ominously now, gathering himself to say something. The older sister suddenly feels her heart flutter. The mother continues staring straight ahead. "I'm sorry to say that it appears likely the cancer has spread," the oncologist says in a low, even tone. "There appear to be some small nodules in your lungs consistent with a diagnosis of metastases. The lungs are among the most common organs to which ovarian tumors spread. We'll have to biopsy the nodules, of course, to make sure our assumptions are correct."

There's silence in the room for an instant. The younger sister then gasps and says, "Dad had lung cancer." The mother continues looking at the doctor, though her eyes are now filling up. The husband puts his hand on his wife's knee. She asks in a shaky voice, "What does this mean? What do we do next?"

The oncologist continues in the same gratingly even tone. "Well, that will depend," he says. "We certainly should do more tests. If they're positive for metastases, then we can consider stronger chemotherapeutic agents. Or we could use radiation therapy to target specific tumors."

Mother is shaking her head now. The older sister notices it and says with alarm, "What, Mom, what?" But the old woman doesn't answer her. The oncologist interrupts, saying, "I'm sure this is a shock. I think we should meet again in a week to talk about all this further. In the meantime, let's set up some additional tests to be clearer about what we're dealing with."

The husband now takes everyone aback by barking angrily, "Is that all the help you can offer us? More tests?" The oncologist looks at him with a studied look of sympathy and says, "There's a lot we can do to improve the quality of your mother-in-law's life. We just need time to come up with the right solutions. I know you're all upset. We'll do all we can to help you." The husband glares at him but says nothing more.

The family moves slowly out of the office, stunned, with a sister on either side holding on to one of Mother's arms and the husband walking with head down a few steps behind them. When they get back to the SUV, the mother seems wrung out and allows her son-in-law to nearly pick her up and place her in the front seat. While driving back to the house, the husband announces suddenly, "It's not a death sentence." The mother turns her face away from him and looks out her side window. The older sister says to him sternly, "Enough. We'll talk about it later."

At home, the mood is at first funereal. Mother and the younger sister sit at the kitchen table with the light off while the older sister busies herself making a pot of tea. The husband drifts back and forth from the kitchen doorway to the basement, unsure whether to sit down and join them. No one talks very much. Finally, the mother, with forced bravado, says, "I'm not hanging crepe, either." The older sister responds immediately, "That-a-girl. Good for you. We'll find out our options. We'll fight this." A few moments later, the older sister walks over to her husband in the hallway outside the kitchen and says, "I think we're all right. Why don't you go to work now?" "You sure?" the husband asks. "Yeah," she answers. "Please go." He feels somewhat reassured but also pushed out. This is female bonding time, and he's in the way. He gathers his files and briefcase from the basement and leaves.

Over the next few days, the older sister is frequently on the basement computer sending and receiving many e-mails. Some of them commiserate; others are for sharing information with her sister, children, and nieces gleaned from various websites about different treatment protocols. By the weekend, grandkids begin to gather in the home, just to sit with Mother at the kitchen table and buoy her up. The great-grandkids are playing on the stairs and running in and out of the kitchen, distracting everyone delightedly. On the living room TV, a baseball game is on, and the only two adult men in the house today, the older and younger sisters' husbands, find themselves gravitating there. While not good friends, after 30 years as brothers-in-law through marriage they've arrived at an easy familiarity. They've been together on the outskirts of these family gatherings many times before.

The game drags. "Real dull," the younger sister's husband pronounces. "The hitters stink," says the older sister's husband. They lapse into quiet again. Then the younger sister's husband asks, "How has everyone been holding up here?"

The older sister's husband replies, "So-so. Mom's not talking much but looks scared. My wife has been even more consumed by all this than she was before. I never see her anymore."

"Oh, yeah," says the younger sister's husband. "We've been through that, too. She's the Queen Worrier," he adds with a nod toward the kitchen to indicate his wife. "But we've had some talks and tried to balance things."

"How have you done that?"

"I just told her she has responsibilities to many people, not just to her mother," says the younger sister's husband. "The longer the cancer goes on, the harder she has to try to make time for all of us."

"Has that worked?"

"Yeah, with some adjustments. It's better now," the younger sister's husband replies. The other man mulls this over while the two of them allow their attention to be drawn to a replay of a double play.

That night, as he's beginning to get ready for bed, the older sister's husband talks himself into and then out of having a conversation with his wife. He badly wants to ask her to find a better "balance" too—one that would include him more in her life. But with the state of mind she's in nowadays there's no telling how she'd react to such a request. He bides his time, reading an old magazine in bed, waiting for her to come up. When she enters the room, she wears a half-smile. "What's up?" he asks her. "Oh, nothing," she says. "Something funny one of the grandkids did." She goes into the bathroom, humming a phrase, and then comes out wearing her pajamas with her hair tied back. He judges she's in the best mood he's seen her in for weeks. "There's something I was hoping to talk with you about," he starts.

"What's that?" she asks.

"Here, why don't you lie next to me," he says. When she sits down on the bed, he adds, "I've been worried."

"Yeah, I've been surprised to see you so worried about Mom," she responds. "That's not usually like you."

"I am worried about your mother," he says, "but I'm also worried about you. And about us."

She looks at him incredulously. "And what does that mean?" she asks.

"You're doing everything you can for your mom," he says in a carefully modulated voice. "It's amazing. But I'm concerned you're wearing yourself out. Plus I never see you anymore. I feel like I'm losing you to the situation."

The older sister looks at him severely for an instant. "I don't need any more pressure," she says. "I'm doing what I feel like I have to do."

He reaches over and puts his hand on her shoulder. "I know, it's very hard," he says. "I want to be able to go through this with you."

"Please take your hand off my shoulder," she orders him. "I'm not in the mood."

He responds, "What?"

"For 35 years," she says calmly, "whenever you've wanted to have sex, you've put your hand on that shoulder. I've been wondering why you've been trying so hard lately to ingratiate yourself with me. But I'm too preoccupied now. It's not the time. You're going to have to wait."

He quickly takes his hand off her shoulder but then protests, "You've got it wrong. This is not about sex. I'm worried."

She springs off the bed, crosses the room, and flicks the light switch off. "Oh, yeah," she says sarcastically in the dark. He feels her bounce back onto the bed, then pull back the sheets and roll over away from him. He lies there, wanting to continue the conversation but afraid of touching or talking to her again. In a few minutes, her shallow breathing suggests she's already fallen asleep. He stares at the ceiling for a while, fuming about what he'll say to her in the morning, and then gives up and closes his eyes.

It's the mission of every family to help all its members sustain themselves through good times and bad. But in a prolonged medical crisis, it isn't unusual for families to (either consciously or unconsciously) direct more resources to helping one family member at other members' expense. In some instances, this can amount to stark economic choices of literally taking the food out of one member's mouth to feed another or spending money on medication for one and not some other member's need. What's more common, however, is for caregiving families to make emotional choices about how they expend their even more valuable resource of intimacy. In its narrowest sense, intimacy refers to physical affection and sex; conceived more broadly, though, it encompasses the time a family devotes to, the attention it lavishes on, and the amount of caring it expresses toward its members. While few caregiving families like to admit they "play favorites," they tend to naturally dote on the ill loved one, who they perceive requires the most help. Think of Charles Dickens's A Christmas Carol: Bob Cratchit, his wife, and their many children rally around Tiny Tim, not only because he's a pure, sweet spirit but because he's lame and vulnerable and needs their extra love.

As with any other family survival strategy, directing the lion's share of intimacy toward one needy member has its pros and cons. In the early stages of a medical crisis or during one that will resolve in weeks or a few months, it makes sense to focus on the member struggling with illness. She'll feel better supported and embrace hope. But especially if the medical crisis goes on for many months or years, the devotion shown to one member may make others experience uncomfortably ambivalent feelings. They may feel jealous and resentful that their own needs aren't being accorded the same attention. They may feel guilty and anxious for even thinking about receiving family concern when a loved one is sick. They may feel deprived and sad that there doesn't seem to be enough intimacy to go around for everyone in the family during the crisis.

Several scenarios suggest that focusing intimacy on one ill member can have potentially negative psychological consequences for others. Imagine, for instance, the healthy older sister of a boy with a severe congenital heart defect. She'll probably take on responsibilities greater than would ordinarily be expected for her age, an experience that will give her an impressive precocious maturity. But she may be so responsive to her sick brother's needs and draw so little attention to her own that she won't fully enjoy a carefree childhood. By the time she's a teenager, she may resent expectations she'll take care of her brother and may begin to rebel, engaging in risky behaviors. As she gets older, she may find herself attracted to men who need her to take care of them, even though such familiar relationships cause her to have powerfully conflicted emotions.

Or consider the young son of a mother with multiple sclerosis. Because "stress" makes her get upset easily, thereby exacerbating her arm and leg weakness, the boy's father pressures him to "behave properly" so his mother won't get worse. The boy tries hard to inhibit his rambunctious nature. As his mother has her inevitable flare-ups during her disease's progression, though, her son has a tendency to blame himself—as if his behavior could really control his mother's illness. He is at risk for becoming a guilt-ridden, depressive boy.

We could also discuss the possibly negative impact on the quality of a marriage of raising a child with cystic fibrosis or taking in a grandparent with advanced chronic obstructive pulmonary disease or having one of the spouses develop severe asthma. We could talk about the loss of family vacations or lack of family attendance at graduations and weddings because one member has acute leukemia or stroke or lupus.

In each of these instances, one member's medical needs take precedence over other members' everyday ones, and the latter suffer to some degree.

If you were the older sister, you might argue that well family members should do what they need to do to care for the member in most pain at the moment; they should suck it up, she would say, and wait their turn to have their own needs met when the crisis abates. But this brings to mind an image of a nest with hungry chicks. If a robin gives worms only to the chick that squawks the loudest, she'll have one thriving bird and the others will perish. Likewise, some family members' needs will go chronically unmet, especially during crises of indefinite duration and indeterminate outcome, and those members will ultimately falter.

To provide ongoing sustenance to all of your kin so they can go forward in life with the greatest success, you must try (as the younger sister's husband suggests) to strike some balance between tending to the neediest relative and taking care of all. You can do that best by making conscious moves to protect and conserve intimacy, doling out nurturance as carefully and justly as possible.

How can you accomplish this? The first step, as always, is raising awareness of the challenge. As discussed in Chapter 4, you and your family members should approach caregiving expecting to make sacrifices that come with assuming new responsibilities, shifting roles, and changing relationships. You should discuss among yourselves how to spread the pain around so it isn't inflicted too severely on one or another relative. By the same token, you should talk about how to share the family's caring, preserving each member's "normal" life as much as possible. Calls to arms to suck it up forever should be rejected. Most of us are neither marines nor martyrs. Everyone deserves a regular break, be it a ballgame, mountain hike, or dinner and a movie. Everybody needs her days of celebration and replenishment. When family members respect your right to have time of your own, that basic consideration and cooperation will help you feel better cared for.

Creating respectful and equitable caregiving arrangements is possible only when communication among family members is open and ongoing. Holding periodic family meetings, either in person or online, is a typical means for relatives to raise awareness of the patient's condition, determine what needs to be done, and then hash out who will take on which tasks and for how long. They frequently also serve as forums for members to inform one another about the demands of their individual lives, ventilate feelings, and express wishes and fears. Just getting together and talking often increases the family's sense of camaraderie in the face of medical threat. This in and of itself implicitly reassures all involved that the family will survive as a loving, caring unit. But these meetings aren't always conflict-free. Sometimes members vie with one another for primary caregiver duties; sometimes they compete at passing the buck. Not every issue gets resolved. So long as everyone is engaged in the negotiations, though, a process is in place to give due consideration to each member's thoughts and feelings. It's a process that should be repeated at regular intervals—such as monthly or quarterly—to review the patient's status and attempt to renegotiate the caregiving plan.

A second step is to strive to keep any family member's need for caring in the context of the whole family. Family psychiatrist Peter Steinglass has often talked about "putting illness in its place." By this he means encouraging a family not to allow medical concerns to become the central enduring drama in its life, but instead to push them toward stage left or right as much of the time as possible. (Better to have illness-related action off-stage altogether, but that's unfortunately not usually in the script.) In other words, providing care to a sick loved one shouldn't subsume all the other characters and plotlines of your family's richer, larger story. With this perspective, other family members' needs for intimacy—raising young children, supporting a struggling marriage, making time for sexual intimacy, and getting through moves and job changes—will never be long shunted from the spotlight and neglected.

If you have a hard time ever shifting the spotlight away from the ill person and her needs, try using the family meeting to make a list of what defines the whole family. What characterizes your clan? What are its main functions? What are the other ongoing needs? What are your values? What events and occasions do you all cherish? What are your hopes for each of the members?

An important aspect of intimacy within families is that it's generally reciprocal. You love your family members, however annoying or maddening they can be, and they love you back despite your faults. One threat to this reciprocity is that the patient becomes a black hole for caring, absorbing all the available love in the family and reflecting back nothing in return. Sometimes this is due to strictly biomedical factors. For example, the ill loved one may be so cognitively impaired because of, say, traumatic brain injury or Alzheimer's dementia that he lacks insight into the magnitude of care he's receiving and lacks the wherewithal to express gratitude or caring in return. These are devastating, as well as extremely depleting, predicaments for family members, who feel the person they loved and who loved them back has vanished, only to be replaced by a bottomless, burdensome pit. Worse, though, is when the patient is cognitively intact but for a variety of psychological reasons—for instance, all-consuming despair, engrossing self-pity, brimming anger, overdependence, and a marauding sense of entitlement—he seems unwilling to appreciate his care. Quite the contrary of expressing loving sentiments, he may even lash out at his caregivers at every opportunity. Family members feel like their intimacy and loyalty have been betrayed in these instances, and, even if they continue caregiving out of filial obligation, they have a hard time suppressing their own hurt and anger. A kind of psychological warfare then often ensues between the bruised but bristling patient and his bedraggled but outraged caregivers.

A third step for protecting intimacy, therefore, is to minimize the loss of mutuality that serious illness frequently causes. As the family caregiver, you need to do more than give care; you need to help devise means for your ill loved one to give care back to you. For example, if your relative no longer has the physical ability to cook dinner, perhaps he should be expected to express thanks and then load the dishwasher afterward. If he can't load the dishwasher, then he can listen intently as you unload about your day's frustrations. If he hasn't the cognitive capacity to listen attentively and understand your emotions, then some other task should be found or created for him. Examples might include sorting the mail and pretending to go through some bills, making the beds, and keeping the kids or grandkids company by watching TV together. Even if you have to go back and redo what he's done or simply check on him, it's worth expending the energy to create the means for him to acknowledge the gift of caring he's received and then return the favor in any way possible. The important thing is that he's expected to make a contribution.

Sometimes caregivers excuse patients from contributing because they either feel guilty holding their poor, sick relative accountable as a responsible family member or find it easier to do all tasks themselves.

This should be avoided for two reasons: Care recipients who are no longer asked to contribute are more likely to become self-centered and demanding or, in contrast, helpless and depressed. Caregivers who neither ask for nor receive acknowledgment or help are more likely to become resentful and burn out. By the same token, caregivers and their ill charges who retain some reciprocal (if unequal) give-and-take are much more successful at preserving intimate bonds; those bonds will make a tremendous difference in how well family members persevere through the medical crisis and afterward.

With these thoughts in mind, we can say that the older sister was on the right track in Chapter 6 when she asked her mother to help out with the family dinner by cutting vegetables. It was a minor gesture, yes, but one designed to slightly remedy how lopsided their relationship had become, bolster the mother's self-esteem, and decrease (in a minor way) the older sister's burden. The older sister should have followed through with her plan, however, and made sure Mother contributed, rather than doing what seemed most expedient by chopping the vegetables herself. By so easily reneging on their agreement, the older sister underscored how little she really needed the mother's help and therefore made her mother feel more worthless than ever. It also may have left the mother with the impression her eldest daughter was lording the position of family matron over her. This could only harm the intimate tie between them.

Three steps to preserving intimacy:

1. Know what caregiving entails and talk about how to spread around the responsibilities.
2. Keep caregiving in perspective—as only one part of the family's story.
3. Make sure the ill family member can give something back.

But the tie that's most strained is the one between the older sister and her husband. On the morning after their tiff, they barely talk to or look at each other. At breakfast, when Mother asks him a question, the husband answers her briefly without raising his eyes from his newspaper. The older sister sees annoyance quickly register on her mother's face. She's about to lay into her husband when he hurriedly removes his dishes from the table with a sulky look and hustles out of the room and down the basement stairs. It serves to confirm the older sister's worst suspicion: He was only being extra nice to her mother recently to get sex. It hurts and disgusts her. Her mother deserves better. She deserves better. Instead, he's behaving like a selfish, manipulative boor. She's tempted to follow him down the steps and give him a piece of her mind but is afraid that, while so angry, she'd only scream at him. Then he'd have an excuse to pout down there for weeks.

The older sister is still straightening up the living room from the previous night's party when the younger sister shows up before lunchtime with cold cuts and fresh rolls. "What's the matter?" the younger sister asks as soon as she walks through the front door and sees her sibling's glower. "I'm sick of doing everything here," the older sister replies grumpily. "Well, that's why I brought lunch," the younger sister responds defensively, waving the plastic deli bag in her hand. The older sister takes the bag from her and begins walking to the kitchen. "I'm not angry at you," she explains over her shoulder. "I'm angry at Bob. He's great at asking for things but not much good at giving."

Accustomed to hearing such griping, the younger sister says nothing as she follows her into the kitchen. The older sister slaps a kettle of water on the stove's front burner to make tea, and the two women sit down at the table. "Where's Mom?" the younger sister asks. "She's upstairs, lying down," the older sister answers and then adds acidly, "The cancer is probably eating her insides and tiring her out." The younger sister grimaces and says, "You're in some mood." "Can you believe," her older sibling asks, "that our mother could be dying and all he thinks about is having sex?" The younger sister pauses before answering, "I don't think Bob is that kind of guy. What are you talking about?" "Why do you think he's been helping out so much recently—like driving us to the doctor's?" argues the older sister. "He feels neglected and sorry for himself and wants me to take care of him like he's some kind of child."

The younger sister pauses again before saying, "Maybe it's not about sex. Maybe he just wants more attention and affection from you. You could be flattered." "What are you talking about?" the older sister shoots back. "For all I've done for him over the years, he has no right to accuse me of anything." She then scrutinizes her sibling and asks, "Has he been talking to you?" The younger sister maintains her calm, stating quietly, "No, he hasn't talked with me. But my own husband talked with me about a month ago. It wasn't very pleasant. He made me aware that Mom's cancer has taken its toll on our relationship. He told me he missed me. I'm sure he wanted to have sex, too, but that wasn't all it was about. He told me I have responsibilities as a wife, not just as a daughter." The older sister doesn't respond, but her face turns slightly flushed. The younger sister goes on, "I don't think what he was saying to me was so wrong. I had gone a little overboard. I needed to rebalance my priorities."

The older sister jumps up to turn off the gas burner. She clatters the tea cups and saucers on the counter. The younger sister braces herself for one of her sibling's tirades, but the older sister merely sits back down and asks her if she wants any honey. The younger sister decides to risk saying more. "What do you think Mother would really want for you?" she asks her. "Even if she was never wild about Bob, do you think she wants you to cut yourself off from him at this point? Do you think Mom thinks that would make you happy?" "Mother doesn't say much about what she's thinking to me," the older sister responds moodily. "She knows I won't cut my husband off. But he needs to back off now so I can concentrate on taking care of her." The younger sister continues in a quieter voice, "And what happens if Mother dies some day? Don't you want your husband close to you then?" The older sister says nothing but glances through the door at the stairway and then stirs her tea vigorously.

No discussion of protecting intimacy in caregiving families would be complete without talking directly about physical intimacy. Whether we are examining the sexual dynamics between ill and well spouses or, as in the case of the older sister and her husband, between frontline caregivers and their spouses, the three steps already outlined—raising awareness of the challenges posed by shifting roles, viewing the patient's needs in the context of the whole family, and minimizing the loss of mutuality—are necessary but not always sufficient for preserving the relationships. With each type of situation, a host of problems frequently curtail any and all physical affection.

In the case of ill and well spouses—a scenario that may be pertinent to your parents if you are caregiving for an aging, ill mother or father—the problems can be biological and/or psychological in complex combinations. For starters, the illness itself can ravage the neurological, hormonal, or vascular underpinnings of the patient's ability to function sexually. In men, this may make maintaining an erection or ejaculating nearly impossible. In women, it may mean the complete loss of libido, vaginal lubrication, or the ability to achieve orgasm. If the disease doesn't cause these sexual problems, then the medications used to treat aspects of the disease—for instance, medicines to lower blood pressure, kill cancer cells, or relieve depression—may alter the body's workings so that sexual dysfunctions are commonplace. Or it may be the combination of disease and its medical treatments that cools the ardor and stymies the person's capacities for lovemaking.

When serious illness holds a family in its grip, the psychological impediments to a couple's sex life are myriad. Foremost among them is blatant fear. When one spouse is recovering from a heart attack or stroke, for example, or declining from a neurological illness such as multiple sclerosis, both spouses are often afraid that sexual activity may exacerbate the disease. It no longer feels like a safe intimate act but instead like a dangerous one, where every soft caress that sends the pulse racing and blood pressure climbing can cause instant medical calamity. Doctors too rarely give couples the education and assurance they need to regain their feeling of security about sex. It often becomes a part of their relationship that, like playing with fire, they shy away from. Ultimately they come to grieve it as lost forever.

A second psychological obstacle is one not unheard of for couples who have never encountered serious illness—performance anxiety. When, because of the disease, medications, or other factors, an ill spouse has an experience of being unable to perform sexually, he may approach future sexual encounters with high anxiety that interferes with his ability to perform again. Unfortunately, multiple occurrences of sexual failure will only make the prospect of physical intimacy so anxiety-inducing that both spouses begin to avoid it to spare each other humiliation and disappointment.

By far, though, the most common barrier to intimacy is the way long-term caregiving changes marital dynamics. Power imbalances are nearly unavoidable. The well spouse, freighted with increased responsibilities, often becomes the dominant adult in the relationship, gradually taking over all decisions. (If she was the dominant one prior to illness, she'll become only more so.) The ill spouse, laden with the indignity of constantly receiving care, frequently regresses to one or another childlike state, either becoming passive and needy or whiny and attention-seeking. Few developments quash the sex life between two loving partners more than the transformation of their emotional relationship into one between an adult and a child. Another way of conceptualizing this is to consider that it's extremely difficult for a well spouse to juggle the roles of nurse and lover. Toileting your husband one moment tends to kill the romantic mood the next. Doing chores all day gives one a passion for sleeping, not frolicking.

There aren't sure-fire answers for these barriers to sex, because every couple has its idiosyncratic issues that must be examined individually. But here are some general suggestions for restoring physical intimacy. If the disease and/or medications are the problem, then medical interventions are essential. Let your doctor guide you toward realistic expectations of sexual functioning at each stage of a disease's progression or recovery. We live in an age when new drugs and treatments for sexual dysfunction are being brought onto the market practically yearly. Your family physician (or a specialist, such as an urologist) ought to be able to offer options for you and your spouse. If medications are the culprit, then alternative drugs or periodic drug holidays should be considered.

Doctors and other healthcare professionals have crucial roles to play in overcoming the psychological barriers, too. The best antidote to fear is education. Simply communicating the medical facts can often allay strong anxiety. Physicians can give spousal caregivers permission to hire help (if financially feasible) to do some of the hands-on care, thereby preserving a woman's duties as a wife rather than as a nurse. They can also give medical blessing to a couple to return to sex; this in and of itself generally provides great relief. Performance anxiety can be treated with patient guidance, the use of erotic movies and sex toys to rekindle libido, and sexual-performance-enhancing medications, such as Viagra.

If it remains a problem, then a form of psychotherapy called sex therapy may be of assistance. Psychotherapy also may be necessary for rebalancing power-skewed marriages. When a disease is disabling and the couple's roles have shifted so drastically that mutuality can't be regained easily, psychotherapists can help couples mourn the previous relationship and attempt to fashion a new connection with its own simple satisfactions.

In the case of frontline caregivers and their spouses, the barriers to sex are a little different. Giving care to an ill loved one expends substantial time and energy. Being busy and fatigued consequently derails caregivers' sex lives (as it does for millions of other overscheduled, sleep-deprived Americans) because they fall into bed each night feeling wiped out, not psyched up. When they say their bedtime prayers, they implore God to give them the energy and patience to get through the next day's ordeals. Extras like sexual fulfillment rarely even enter their thoughts.

Resentment and guilt are other obstacles every bit as difficult. When caregivers have embraced the spartan ethic of providing intensive around-the-clock care, they may experience their spouses' requests for sex as nearly otherworldly. Worse, they may resent those requests as somehow detracting from the pursuit of their mission—that is, having fun sexually is incompatible with focusing mentally on saving an ill loved one. For those whose caregiving commitments have not consumed them to the same extent, engaging in sexual activity when a loved one is sick may provoke strong guilt—as if their pleasure would somehow trivialize their ill relative's suffering or add to his pain. They may consequently block a spouse's repeated sexual advances as a means of avoiding harsh self-criticism, even if it means risking damage to their own marriage.

If there's anything we've learned during the past decade from renowned marriage researchers such as John Gottman, it's that spouses whose interactions aren't largely positive are at high risk for divorce. You must continue to talk, share, and have fun with your spouse or witness the demise of intimacy, possibly irreparably. There's no putting off investing time and energy into a marriage until after a prolonged medical crisis is over, because the viability of that marriage may be severely damaged. Even if you only talk with your spouse for 20 minutes a day (the amount of time research suggests the average noncaregiving couple actually converse), you need to connect emotionally during that time through cuddling, confiding, and commiserating to keep the loving friendship alive. Even if feelings of resentment and guilt plague you, talk about them with your spouse (for example, "Can I raise something that's troubling me?"). At least he'll then be in the emotional loop and may even help assuage those uncomfortable feelings. If that's not possible without spurring a negative reaction from him, then perhaps it's time to attend a support group or make an appointment with a professional counselor to better manage those emotions. It does no one any good to caregive heroically and, in the process, let your marriage die from poor tending.

That night, it's the older daughter who nervously waits in bed with a magazine for her spouse to come upstairs. She hasn't made up her mind about what she'll say to him. She has no intention of apologizing. For what purpose? she reasons. But her younger sister's admonitions have left her uneasy. No matter how mad she is at him, she doesn't want to alienate him. It may be a good idea to at least open the channels of communication.

Her husband soon comes into the room, a tight look of simmering anger on his face, and strides past her toward the bathroom without greeting her. She feels herself getting annoyed when he takes an extra long time flossing and brushing, running the water full blast continuously. When he finally comes out, she still feigns reading her magazine as he settles onto the far side of his half of the king-sized bed. She says nonchalantly after a few moments, "How was your day?" He reacts by giving her a startled stare before quickly looking away and flipping on the television with the remote control. She waits a few moments and then says firmly, "Please turn off the TV." After ignoring her for a few seconds, he clicks the television off and turns his head to face her.

"All right. All right, already," she blurts out. "So, I got angry with you last night, and now you're being angry back."

"That is *not* why I'm angry with you," he says.

"Yeah, we're not spending enough time together," she says in a singsong that verges on sarcasm.

"Don't start again about sex," her husband says with his voice rising.

She quickly changes her tone to a more serious one, saying, "You're concerned we're not spending enough time together."

"You make it sound like a small thing," he replies, still furious. "It's not a small thing. You don't seem to get that."

The older daughter pauses and then reaches out and rests her hand on her husband's shoulder. "What am I supposed to do?" she asks in a tired voice. "My mother is sick and needs me. I expected that you'd understand that. I guess I was mistaken." She sighs and adds, "I know we haven't seen much of each other."

He's so exasperated that he pulls his shoulder away from her hand and fumes silently, staring up at the ceiling. After a few moments, he says in his own weary voice, "I do understand you want to take care of your mom. I really want to support you in that. But I don't want to be cut off from you also. Of course I want to have sex with you, but what I miss most is hanging around and talking. What is so terrible about that?"

"It's not so terrible," she responds in a quieter, more conciliatory voice. "I have a lot to do all the time. I miss you, too."

They lie there looking up at the ceiling without speaking for a minute. The husband then asks in a hesitant, little-boy voice, "Can we make a regular time to spend together without having to take care of your mother?" The older daughter muses on this for an instant before answering, "That's fine. Maybe something weekly. I'll get my sister to help." But then she adds, "Can you make the commitment to helping out with Mom on a more regular basis so everything doesn't fall on my shoulders?"

He shifts around in the bed, rolling flat on his back. "Yeah, I can do that," he murmurs. He then reaches out and touches her shoulder and she gives a little start. She says in a pressured tone: "My mother is down the hall full of cancer. I want to be close to you, but I'm not ready to make love with you. Please be patient with me."

Her husband withdraws his arm and says with resignation, "Okay, okay." Pushing himself into a sitting position against the headboard, he grabs the remote control and once again flicks the TV on.

Preserving the sanctity of loving relationships is an essential challenge for those who've committed to giving care. Even more crucial, however, are efforts to preserve a sense of the sanctity of everyday life. Spirituality and religion are means of finding hope in the world when despair over a serious illness colors all thoughts about the family's present and future. In the next chapter, we'll explore means of sustaining spirituality in the face of heart-rending medical decline.

Can a Spouse Be Nurse and Lover Too?

Q: *My mother's physical disability requires Dad to help her with a lot of daily physical functions, from toileting to dressing and getting in and out of bed and her wheelchair. Until Mom's illness, I had always thought of the two of them as very active, lively senior citizens who did pretty much everything much younger people did. I suppose that included sex, though I never gave it any thought until recently, when Mom started making cryptic comments to me about "life" not having to end between her and Dad just because she spends much of her day in a wheelchair. She seems very hurt by the change in my dad, though she doesn't give me any details and I don't feel comfortable asking. But I hate to see a rift developing between them when they have so much else to deal with. Is there anything I can do to help?*

A: I've seen countless couples whose sex lives diminish, if not altogether disappear, as caregiving comes to dominate their lives. This is especially true for those marriages in which the ill spouse needs hands-on care. The causes are many. One of the key reasons is that intensive caregiving often changes the balance within relationships from that of equal partners to one-sided arrangements in which mutuality, a primary ingredient of sexual intimacy, is lost. Few of us would feel comfortable making love to our spouses if the dynamics of our marriage had evolved into those between a parent and child. Another reason is that the emotionally detached task orientation that many caregivers adopt to get through providing arduous hands-on care makes it more difficult for them to feel sexually intimate. Also, it's nearly impossible to act as a nurse one moment—a different type of intimacy—and switch to the role of lover the next. A third reason is more mundane but probably the most influential of all: Hands-on caregivers are often too darn tired from their daily grind to even think about having sex.

For your parents to avoid a widening emotional and physical rift between them, much depends on what each of them wants. Do they want to adapt to a new relationship in which sex plays little or no role, or do they want to reintroduce sex into their lives? Do both of them want the same thing?

If they both want to reclaim their sexual relationship, it will take passion to rekindle any conjugal sparks. First and foremost, they'll need to restore as much balance in their relationship as possible so that your father regards your mother as more of a partner who helps him than a patient he takes care of. Maybe your dad avoids discussing the problem with her because he's afraid he'll hurt her feelings, but his silence will only increase your mother's doubts about herself. Dad needs to treat her as a full-fledged adult with whom he can converse about a very difficult subject so that his wife has the opportunity to advise him and the two of them can face the problem together. Talking openly and intimately about their lack of sex life may, somewhat paradoxically, bring the two of them emotionally closer and create conditions for increased physical affection.

If talking alone doesn't better balance their relationship and increase their intimacy, they might consider a more radical step if they can afford it: Minimize the amount of hands-on care your dad does by hiring a home health aide to do the dirty work. By that means, your father will better preserve his primary role as doting husband, rather than dutiful nurse, to your mom. That may yet awaken old stirrings in him that have been dormant during these years of having to get things done.

In truth, I've seen many couples get caught up in the rigors of caregiving and give up on their sex lives; those who try to resurrect physical intimacy often struggle. Yet I think of Marvin Gaye's classic

"Sexual Healing" as a paean to the power of lovemaking to salve all wounds. Disabled and disheartened care receivers need that. Duty-bound caregivers do too. You may need to help your parents find a counselor, whether a therapist or a clergyperson, to help them through this problem.

Giving Care Does Not Include Taking Abuse

Q: *My father, who lives with me, suffered a stroke recently, and his personality has changed dramatically. He has become verbally abusive, and I'm afraid the verbal abuse might turn physical. I want to be there for him, but I don't know how much more I can take. He feels like a total stranger to me. What can I do?*

A: What could be more demoralizing than to be castigated or even threatened by a family member to whom you've devoted yourself? There may be specific means, though, of understanding and curtailing your father's behavior and assuring your safety. Before giving up on caregiving, there are neurological and psychological interventions to consider.

Patients who suffer brain damage from a slowly progressing disease, such as Alzheimer's dementia, or a sudden event, such as a head trauma or stroke, often experience changes not only in overall personality but in specific cognitive functions, including emotional expressiveness, self-control, capacity for insight into their own deficits, and ability to empathize with others. For example, a rule of thumb with stroke victims is that those who've had damage to the left side and frontal regions of their brains are usually more depressed afterward. Those with right-sided damage may be more emotionally inexpressive (what doctors call "flat") or prone to sudden shifts in emotions (called "lability"), including vicious tirades. While some of these symptoms may disappear along with other stroke-induced problems (for example, difficulties with walking, talking, and swallowing) over 6 months or more, many patients will be left vastly different people than they were before the medical cataclysm struck.

I strongly recommend conferring about your father's behavior with his neurologist, psychiatrist, or, best yet, neuropsychiatrist (a physician who specializes in the behavioral and mood changes due to neurological problems). He or she may prescribe a low dose of an atypical anti-psychotic medication, such as Risperdal, to better control his agitation and decrease his outbursts. Or the doctor may subscribe to the old adage that "anger is depression turned outward" and give your father an antidepressant to ease his frustrations and allay his attacks on you. Such drug interventions are frequently successful in these kinds of cases.

Counseling may also be helpful if conducted by a therapist conversant with relationship issues common among the neurologically impaired. Your father may gain greater awareness of his frustrations and insight into the hurtful impact of his words and actions. You may glean particular strategies for setting limits with him. For instance, you may learn to avoid specific stressors—for example, loud noises, crowds of people—that, reasonably or not, seem to stoke his ire. You may also learn to cue him when you note his frustrations rising so he can begin to exert greater control over his impulses. Finally, you can be coached to firmly say to him you won't tolerate verbal abuse and will leave the room or house if he persists.

Fortunately, verbal abuse isn't necessarily a harbinger of physical abuse. However, if your father should ever lay a hand on you, throw things at you, or—heaven forbid—wield a weapon in your direction, your first duty is to protect yourself. Leave and get help. Call the police if need be. Caregivers are not whipping posts. You're not required to take punches while giving love.

A Daughter Distanced by Family Change

Q: *Since my father severely herniated a disk in his neck over a year ago, our family life has changed dramatically. He has lived with me and my 17-year-old daughter since she was 3, when my husband died, and he's been more like a father to her than a grandfather. Now he's had to cut back his electrician's job to part-time status and has gotten very moody and self-absorbed hanging around the house. I've had to go back to work to make up for the shortfall in his income. I'm worried these changes have had a bad effect on my daughter. She and her grandfather hardly talk anymore but often just ignore each other. She's also hard for me to get through to. I'd like to improve our relationships before she goes off to college next year. What can I do?*

A: It's natural for older teenagers to be more involved with their friends, jobs, and favorite activities than they are with their own families. It's a way for them to prepare themselves emotionally for separating from their parents when they move away to college. But this distancing process usually takes place gradually over a number of years. If your daughter suddenly stopped talking with you and her grandfather around the time he injured his neck, her aloofness is probably a product, at least in part, of her reaction to the family's medical ordeal. Her behavior might reflect her sadness about how the family has changed and how you (because of working) and her grandfather (because of self-absorption) are less attuned to her needs. It's also plausible that she's angry at her grandfather for how he's handled his partial disability. Maybe she's also mad at him for not having taken good enough care of himself to avoid becoming injured. Maybe she's mad at you for not having made him rest more and take better care of his body.

There are four potential ways to approach her. One is to simply leave her be and wait her out. She'll eventually mature, better adjust to the changed family circumstances, and accept that her elders are flawed people, vulnerable to illness and to moodiness and unhealthy lifestyle habits at times. But this will likely take years, all the longer because of her absence from your home while at college. If there's unfinished family business, it's preferable to address it before she goes.

A second strategy would be to encourage your daughter and father to spend more time together and figure out how to relate to each other better. Perhaps they could even rekindle interests they previously had shared. The likelihood is, though, they'd both resist it. Time doesn't flow backward, and neither does development. Your daughter has moved on from her interests of several years ago, and her grandfather is also a different person. They'd have to discover or create some new commonalities. That will be hard so long as they're mostly bristling at each other.

A third approach would be for you to make concerted efforts to spend time alone with her. She may resist this, too, but I'd insist on it. The key question to discuss with her is this: How has she been affected by the many changes that have occurred in the family over the past year? Unless she's especially articulate for her age and accustomed to expressing her feelings, she initially may not respond much to this question at all. You may have to come back to it again and again or even suggest various emotions she may be having: Is she sad to see her grandfather having such difficulties? Is she angry at him for acting self-centeredly at times? Is she worried he might injure himself further and become even more disabled? Is she glad to be away from the house most of the time so she doesn't have to think about the family's medical and money problems? If she continues to have trouble expressing how she feels but you sense that she's feeling a great deal, you may consider getting her an individual psychotherapist to help her sort out her emotions so they don't impede her relationships or aspirations.

I think the best solution, however, would be a fourth one—having all of you speak with a neutral party about what's occurred to you individually and as a family. Even at a time when your daughter may desire greater distance from you and your father, the ways you act toward her are going to affect how she feels. Perhaps family therapy, as an adjunctive treatment to her individual counseling, could help you grieve together about what you've all lost since the injury and begin to talk together about what you each need to grow and thrive at this time. Her grandfather needs to hear how the manner in which he handles his partial disability has repercussions for the rest of the family. Your daughter needs to realize that she has the power to make the family's interactions go better or worse depending on her degree of acceptance and accommodation. You can learn how to draw everyone closer now so that it'll be easier to let your daughter go away to college in a year without the encumbrance of so much old anger and pain.

Reclaiming a Sister Lost to Caregiving

Q: *My sister and I are only 18 months apart in age and have always been best friends. We're fortunate that, as adults, our families settled in the same town and we're able to see each other almost every day. But in the past year, we haven't seen each other nearly that much since my sister's father-in-law had a heart attack. I understood during the first few months afterward that she felt she had to spend a lot of time helping with his recovery—he lives alone and depends on my sister and her husband. But his condition has been stable for some time now, and yet she still feels like she has to hover over him. I miss her and am also mad at her. How do I convince her to make room for me in her life again?*

A: Anger won't restore your closeness with your sister; renewed empathy might. I'd keep in mind that heart attacks have a way of making victims feel suddenly mortal and loved ones feel terrified. Those emotions often persist for years. It's not unusual that your sister still feels the need to watch over her father-in-law, especially if she is particularly close to him and/or she is following her husband's lead, as if through her oversight she can ward off further calamity. Perhaps she took her father-in-law for granted prior to his heart attack and consequently feels guilty that her relative lack of attention to his diet, exercise, and overall health made him susceptible to death and her husband vulnerable to being orphaned. She probably has no intention of taking that risk again. It's not that she wants to neglect you, but she's still seeking a way of handling her anxiety about her father-in-law while attending to the rest of her life.

My strongest advice, therefore, is not to oppose her focus on her father-in-law but to find ways of joining her in her urgent mission. Become her confidante about her concerns about his health. Share heart-healthy recipes with her. Go for walks with her and her husband and father-in-law. Make sure your sister realizes you're her biggest ally and fan.

Only then would I consider broaching the subject that you've missed her over the past year. Tell her how much you love her and how important she is to you. Explain that you have no desire to come between her and her husband and his family but you'd like to see her more. If she responds defensively, as if you're making her feel guilty, immediately back off by telling her you'll be happy to see her whenever she feels able to make the time. If she's receptive to your entreaties, make regular plans that won't conflict with times her husband and father-in-law may need her. Be sure to express your willingness to accommodate her by changing those plans whenever duty to her husband's family calls.

In all likelihood, if her father-in-law's medical condition continues to be stable, your sister will gradually gain more confidence that her life and her husband will be all right. As her anxiety slowly decreases, she probably will be more spontaneous and flexible in attending to all of her relationships. She may even thank you one day for having been so supportive during this prolonged crisis period in her life.

CHAPTER EIGHT

Sustaining the Spirit

Before dawn, the mother's eyes involuntarily flutter open, and she wakes suddenly as if she's heard someone crying out. In the silence that follows, she lies there in a state of confusion about whether the high-pitched wail came from someone else or from her. Then doubts that there was a sound at all begin to collect in her foggy mind. Little difference it makes, she grumbles. It's the ninth or tenth morning in a row in which, for whatever reason, she's been awakened in the dark much earlier than she wants. Frustrated, she spends the next hour staring at the shadows of tree branches becoming sharper on the yellowed shade in her granddaughter's room as the sun rises. Her mind becomes sharper too, focusing on one specific worry after another—her recent test results, her upcoming chemotherapy (called "more aggressive" by her oncologist), her mysteriously swollen legs. She hadn't been surprised a week ago when the needle biopsy confirmed the nodules in her lung were metastases of her ovarian cancer. She'd even been aware (or maybe just imagined?) she was slowly becoming shorter of breath. And what about her legs? Were they puffy with fluid trickling down from her lungs? No one has told her so, but as she moves them back and forth beneath her blankets, she wonders if cancer cells have somehow taken residence in them too.

Her legs remind her a little of her father's toward the end of his life. His were stout and hairy, like shaggy-barked tree trunks, swollen from gout, she thinks, or perhaps congestive heart failure; she was never sure. And then, without thinking, an old melody her father used to sing—part-hymn, part-children's rhyme—arises from the depths of her memory, a few words at first and then all at once:

> The sun comes up
> The grass shines with dew
> God has made His plans
> For a brighter day for you

It was a silly ditty he had crooned in a scratchy voice as he stroked her hair at bedtime when she was very young. She didn't know where he'd learned it or whether he'd made it up for her. He was a poorly educated immigrant, a tender-hearted working man, who was never well versed in church teachings but who held to the conviction that God watches over and protects us. The song captured that basic belief so simply, she reasons, he must have made it up. She can't recall the last time the tune had occurred to her—maybe as long as 70 years ago, when she became old enough to tuck herself into bed. She doesn't know why it would return now but feels better just thinking about the soothing effect it had when she used to have trouble settling down to sleep. She repeats the words to herself and then tries to remember the rest of the lyrics and the tired look on her father's face as he chanted them. Nothing else comes to her mind, though.

Her thoughts return to the words she remembers. She wonders, What plans has God made for me? Though her minister had advised her the last time she was in the hospital to calm her mind by "leaving all cares in God's hands," she is by temperament too controlling and by experience too mistrustful to do that easily. Instead, the question of God's plans has vexed her repeatedly in recent days, particularly in the dim early hours. It has led her down two tracks of spiritual thought that run parallel at times, crisscross at others, without reaching any satisfying end.

The first track disturbs her. During these restless mornings, she has kept casting her mind back over her life in an attempt to understand why God would punish her. She admits she's been no Holy Roller. She never liked the fancy airs people put on in church; she'd go only on Christmas, Easter, and the odd Sunday to sit quietly in some back pew. But she's always had good moral values. And she's devoted herself to her children and grandchildren, making sure they go to church regularly. God knows she was a good wife, even during the agonizing days of her husband's illness. She is grateful for the good life she's had. But old age's pains, worries, and loss of independence are not what she considers to be just rewards for a lifetime of integrity.

The second track is more distressing. She has come to question how God could make anyone suffer with cancer. What could be a more horrible end, she shudders, than being devoured from the inside by one's own frenzied cells? Who could deserve it? How could she leave her cares in God's hands while knowing He tortures people so? She's strong enough in her faith not to deny God's existence but is enough of a skeptic to doubt His judgment and purpose. Questions about that purpose nag at her during the long hours she lies in bed, angering and even sickening her. On the few Sunday mornings her older daughter has come upstairs to invite her to church with her, the mother has answered simply, "I can't bring myself to go yet."

This morning she finds herself reverting to an old habit—talking out loud to God about her doubts about God. She says idly, "Show me something—anything." The first part of the sentence is said in an emotionless tone as if she doubts the prospect of seeing any sign. But when she pronounces the word "anything," her voice has a note of yearning, of fervor, that suggests she wants to believe in heaven-sent portents. She lifts her head off the pillow and glances around the room as if waiting. She then lowers her head back down and turns her face to one side, muttering "Ridiculous." But as the word leaves her mouth, she feels a pang of guilt. Perhaps, she chides herself, it's arrogant of her to even ask for a sign, as if God were a magician doing tricks on command. To make amends, she begins quickly reciting The Lord's Prayer under her breath, then rolls over and stares at the wall. She lies there for a long time, feeling sad and empty. "Enough already. Get up," she finally says out loud to herself while slowly pulling back the blanket and awkwardly swinging her legs over the side of the bed.

She crosses the room unsteadily to get a clean house dress out of the closet. She can hear her older daughter stomping around downstairs. As she slips the dress over her head, she notes that her arms are stiff and her lower back is aching. "Quit moping," she whispers to herself. To brighten her mood, she goes over to the window, lifts up the shade, and allows the morning sunshine to stream into the room. She squints as she looks up at the sky to see what the weather will be for the day. She then directs her gaze downward to see if the morning paper is lying on the walkway. Glancing at the front lawn, she has to squint again because of the bright sheen. The thought hits her as powerfully as a revelation: The grass is shining with dew. Her heart suddenly beats hard in her chest, and she feels her lips curling back into an open-mouthed look of joy and astonishment. "God did hear my prayers," she exclaims in a loud voice. "Or was it my loving father watching over me?" she asks herself in the next moment. The sunlight feels warm on her face like fresh hope for her future.

Hope during a medical crisis comes in many forms. We place our trust in the surgeon's knife, the internist's pills, and the oncologist's deadly arsenal or have faith in the character and know-how of the doctors wielding them. We believe our bodies somehow intuit how to heal. We expect family and friends to bolster us. But when we exhaust biomedical solutions and the support of our closest companions, most of us turn to powers beyond this earthly realm. Many explicitly call on prayer and personal relationships with God; others draw from spiritual notions of the energies in the universe. We ask for healing. When healing is not possible, we beseech the higher powers to give us understanding and acceptance of our condition.

Religious and spiritual disciplines have always linked espousals of faith to improved health. The first healthcare workers were shamans who conducted religious rituals, induced trance states, and dispensed herbs and potions to dispel evil spirits. Physicians from the 18th and 19th centuries, whether in the hospital, office, or patient's home, routinely ministered to body and soul. But as scientific advances revolutionized medicine in the 20th century, redefining physicians as masters of technology-based tests and treatments, the patient's spirit received less attention. Especially in the past 50 years, doctors stuck largely to observing somatic symptoms and devising biomedical interventions. Nurses, social workers, and psychologists attended to patients' emotional states but only occasionally to their religious needs. While ministers, priests, and rabbis continued to come to hospital rooms to pray with their seriously ill congregants, they were relegated to being helpful after-hours visitors rather than central players on the healthcare team.

In the past two decades, numerous factors have created a renewed interest in spirituality and health. Most are reactions to what many people have perceived as the sterility of modern technological medicine. In the past 30 years, authors such as Lawrence LeShan and Bernie Siegel have published popular self-help books for cancer patients that urged them to depend on the power of positive attitudes, meditation, and self-determination and not simply the godlike commandments of their oncologists. At the same time, the hospice movement, emphasizing acceptance and spiritual values at the end of patients' lives, became more widespread in this country. More recently, so-called alternative, complementary, or integrative approaches to health, using natural remedies, stress management, and heightened spiritual awareness, have gained popularity among Americans who are doubtful about physicians' reliance on costly tests and side effect-inducing pharmaceutical drugs. The result has been a veritable cultural shift in how we safeguard health. There are, for example, now literally hundreds of thousands of websites and tens of thousands of books and magazines available on using spirituality to promote wellness. Also, several recent surveys have found that the majority of patients want their doctors to ask them about their spiritual and religious lives.

The medical community hasn't been immune to these cultural changes. Within the past 10 years, concerted efforts have been made in several quarters to integrate greater understanding of patients' spiritual and religious beliefs into biomedicine. This is seen most clearly in three significant developments. The first concerns changes in clinical practice. Many major medical institutions have set up integrative medical centers that incorporate stress management and religious practices into traditional biomedical care. Most hospital-run hospice programs have included chaplains as part of their care teams. And mainstream medical journals, including *The Journal of Family Practice*, have published articles in recent years with such titles as "Principles to Make a Spiritual Assessment in Your Practice." These articles attempt to guide physicians in the art of asking patients about their spiritual beliefs without causing offense or unduly influencing those views.

The second development involves curricular changes in medical education. Most American medical schools now have lectures and courses to help budding physicians solicit and harness patients' spiritual views. Some go further to help fledgling doctors reflect on how their own spiritual beliefs affect their views of patients, diseases, and practicing the healing arts.

Third and perhaps most important—in an age when empirical evidence has become the gold standard for guiding clinicians in their selections of patients' treatments—large research centers have now taken up the study of the healing potential of spirituality. The National Institutes of Health, through the National Center for Complementary and Alternative Medicine, is now funding (at least on a modest scale) research into the impact of patients' religious and spiritual beliefs and practices on medical outcomes. Academic research centers on the topic have been established at Duke University, George Washington University, and the University of Florida.

In the 2001 book *Handbook of Religion and Health*, Duke University professor Harold Koenig reviewed 1,600 research studies and grouped them into religion and mental health, religion and physical disorders, and religion and the use of health services. Studies in the first category found that people who regularly attended a church, synagogue, or mosque had fewer episodes of depression, lower rates of drug and alcohol use, and better capacity for coping with illness and other stressors. Studies in the second category linked spirituality with lower blood pressure, cholesterol levels, and mortality rates, as well as improved immune function. The third category's research suggested people with strong spiritual beliefs were more likely to use health prevention services (for example, annual checkups, mammograms) and to follow doctors' instructions. While these results represent early steps of a growing effort that requires more study, they support the idea that religious activity and beliefs can be powerful tools for the ill. (To read examples of abstracts of research studies on spirituality and health, you can peruse the excellent website for the Duke Center for Spirituality, Theology and Health at www.dukespiritualityandhealth.org.)

But, as with most subjects in life, the impact of spirituality on health is complex. Some of the Duke studies indicate certain religious activities and beliefs can actually be harmful to health. For example, one research project, done in part at Duke but principally authored by Kenneth Pargament, PhD, of Bowling Green University, found that people who believed in God but thought He was punishing them or had abandoned them when they were sick (so-called negative coping) had significantly higher mortality rates. Findings such as this suggest the impact of spirituality is likely beneficial for certain people under specific circumstances but not always so for others.

This is borne out as well in a dilemma commonly discussed in biomedical ethics classes. Particular religious persuasions prohibit their followers from accepting blood transfusions or permitting surgical treatments. These people are no doubt strengthened by their faith. Yet, their religious practices may place them at odds with physicians' recommendations; in an emergency, they may decline life-saving medical measures for themselves or their children. When such cases come before the courts, rulings have consistently supported proceeding with life-saving interventions even if they violate patients' religious convictions. But no clinician is entirely comfortable administering a treatment against a patient's or parent's will. When spirituality creates adversarial relationships between the ill and their healthcare providers, it can only be regarded as a mixed blessing.

> Many people turn to spirituality during a medical crisis, but research shows that it can be a mixed blessing. A lot depends on the attitude you bring to it. Do you and your relative gain understanding and acceptance of the illness you're dealing with when you turn to your religion or a higher power? Or do you feel you're being punished? Do you take comfort in returning to a house of worship if you haven't been actively religious, or does it feel hypocritical to do so only when life gets hard?

Other factors complicate our assessment of spirituality's benefit. Not least among them is that there isn't universal agreement about what spirituality is. Some commentators say it involves the presence of a higher power (as in Alcoholics Anonymous) or a god (as in religions). They differ in their opinions about how best to connect with that presence—through prayer (Western religions) or meditation (Eastern religions) or contemplation of nature (Romantic poetry) or even endorphin-rich feats of physical endurance (for example, the transcendent "runner's high"). They all posit, though, that achieving connection with that higher power provides a sense of peace, wholeness, and well-being that's especially important for people who are faced with difficult challenges such as serious illness.

Others see spirituality in more secular terms—as the pursuit of the state of peace and wholeness itself without necessarily involving the presence of any god. For example, in its section on "Spirituality and Health" on familydoctor.org, the American Association of Family Physicians' medical information website, spirituality is defined very broadly as "the way you find meaning, hope, comfort and inner peace in your life." Its pathways can be as various as doing breathing exercises, contemplating one's values and principles, writing, praying, sewing, and so on. Practice is the key here; belief in a higher power is optional. The website states that many of us who are ill or troubled can benefit from having such spiritual means of calming ourselves in the face of suffering and debilitation.

Yet, other people feel embracing God-centered or godless spirituality during a medical crisis is hypocritical if they never lived by those values previously. For every 10 people who embrace religion when they become fearful that they or their loved ones are going to die, there's probably one person who resists the calling, turns down the offer to talk with the hospital chaplain, and goes stony silent when others insist on praying for her. She may turn aside the entreaties of the hospital social worker as well and eschew recommendations for breathing exercises or stress management, saying those aren't the ways she's chosen to cope. She may keep a stiff upper lip and be stoic and try very hard not to let doubts about God, eternity, or turns of fate enter her mind. But, frequently, those doubts have ways of arising unbidden anyway.

On a bright, quiet Sunday morning, the younger daughter heads her car into the city with hopes of taking her mother out for brunch. By slipping out while her sister is at church, she won't have to compete for Mother's attention as she does whenever the three of them are together. But as she pulls into her sister's driveway, she's greeted by her brother-in-law, pushing a hand-mower through the tall grass, who tells her that her sister and mother should be back from church soon. The younger daughter is startled. What would prompt Mother to attend services now, she wonders, when she hasn't gone in many months? After her brother-in-law waves her into the house, she puts a kettle of water on the stove for tea and takes a seat at the kitchen table to wait impatiently for them to return.

She feels annoyed for several reasons. Certainly she's disappointed she isn't going to see her mother alone. But she also resents her sister for likely pressuring Mom to go to church today. As she turns the heat off under the whistling kettle, though, she reconsiders this assessment. Her sister has never been able to coerce their mother into going before. Perhaps Mom decided on her own to attend services this morning. Anxious thoughts then cross the younger daughter's mind: Is today the anniversary of some important loss—Dad's succumbing to cancer or her mother's mother's death? If so, Mom would have wanted to go to church to light a candle. She then questions, however, if it isn't a time of remembrance at all but instead a time to ask for special healing. Has her mother had some further medical setback she hasn't told her about? The younger daughter is positive her mother and sister don't tell her everything; they think she's too sensitive. What would that setback be if Mother were having one? She already has metastases; what could be worse? Agitated now, the younger daughter gets up and starts pacing the linoleum floor.

What doesn't occur to her is the possibility her mother has chosen to go out of a desire to pray alongside other congregants in a stained-glass-tinted, incense-tinged house of worship. That's not the mother she knows, who has always said she doesn't need a high-collared pastor or soaring steeple to have a talk with God; she could do it in the humble kitchen or bedroom of her own house just as well. It's also not how the younger daughter thinks about her own spirituality. Like many people who've lost loved ones to serious illness, the younger daughter was furious at God after her father died in terrible pain. She refused to go back to church for years, even at her mother's behest. She couldn't understand how her older sister simply went on attending services as if nothing unjust or catastrophic had happened. Eventually, the younger daughter did go back, accompanying her mother to Easter services one year, Christmas Eve services the next. But something had gone out of her engagement with organized religion. She felt a stronger sense of a higher power while walking her dog in the woods by her house or standing by the bedside at the birth of her grandchild. She can deal with that kind of God—the miracle-of-being sort—not the austere, rule-bound Lord of the church. She no longer believes her dad is in heaven but that he's just gone—bones and teeth in a box in the ground to eventually be reabsorbed into the circle of life.

In reality, the younger daughter would judge herself a hypocrite if she were to go back to church regularly. She can't exactly blame Mother if she gravitates toward religion at a time of crisis in her life but would be surprised by it. No, to be truthful to herself, she would have to admit it probably would upset her. She's always admired her mother for living life on her own terms and not giving a hoot about what other people say or do. Embracing formal religious doctrines and rituals would be out of character for her. To the younger daughter, that would be like her mother giving up on who she's been.

After a while, the younger daughter hears a car pull up, then a door slamming hard and then another one more lightly. Her mother's walker makes a dull clinking sound as she places it down in the driveway gravel. The younger daughter sits back down and tries to compose herself. She wants no big scene on a pleasant Sunday morning. The older sister comes in first and says matter-of-factly, "Oh, you're here. Is there enough hot water for us?" Mother follows her in with a look of fatigue but contentment. "I'll put up more water," the younger daughter responds and carries the kettle over to the sink. "Isn't Mom looking well?" the older sister asks. "She did so well at church." "That's great," says the younger daughter in a small voice. "We both enjoyed the sermon," the older sister continues. "It was about trusting in God even through adversity." The younger daughter feels her face reddening. She has the distinct impression her sister is hinting she should just get over whatever it is that's troubling her and come back to church regularly with them. She and her sister have had arguments about this before, and she has no desire to repeat them today. She makes no reply; the older sister drops the subject. Mother, too, says nothing.

They are drinking their tea in silence, and the mother is picking at a plate of tuna salad when the brother-in-law comes in to ask the older sister for a hand with straightening up outside. The older sister gets up and leaves without finishing her tea. The younger daughter immediately takes the opportunity to grill her mother. "I'm glad you enjoyed church this morning," she says. "I didn't realize you were going. I had come by to take you out to brunch."

"Oh, that's too bad," the mother replies. "I would have enjoyed going with you. You should have called first."

It isn't the younger daughter's intention to bemoan the missed brunch. "So what made you go this morning? You haven't been in ages," she says quickly.

"No real reason," the mother responds in the same quiet tone. "Your sister asked me, and I thought it would be nice."

"Did she push you to go?" the younger daughter immediately questions her.

"Not at all," the mother insists. "I wanted to go."

The younger daughter doesn't let up. "It's just that it's not like you," she says. "I hope nothing's wrong."

"To the contrary," the mother says, "there's more right now than before."

"What do you mean?" her daughter asks.

The mother is quiet for several moments, running her fork around the edges of the tuna salad. "I don't want you to get the wrong idea," she says. "It's not something I can explain easily." She is silent again for a long pause as her daughter waits anxiously. Mother begins again suddenly, saying rapidly, "I had a sign from God—or maybe it was your father—that they're watching over me and things are going to go better for me. I thought the least I can do in return is go to church and pay my respects to them."

The younger daughter is flabbergasted. "What sign?" she asks.

"It's not important," says the mother. "In fact it might sound silly to you, but it meant something to me."

The daughter asks, "Did you hear voices?"

"No, I didn't hear voices," the mother responds forcefully. "Do you really think I'm that far gone? I think you can have some sense of God without being crazy."

Now it's the daughter who's silent. She stares out the kitchen window, trying to imagine what her mother could have experienced. She doesn't know what to make of it or what to say. Should she congratulate her mother or fear for her sanity? (Maybe Mom has metastases on her brain, making her hallucinate.) Is her revelation a good thing or bad? She doesn't want to come across as critical. But before she has the time to formulate a proper response, her mother speaks to her again.

"You're entitled to your beliefs, and I'm entitled to mine," she says defensively. She then adds as an afterthought, "Your sister took it in stride."

The younger daughter feels stung. To protest now would make her only seem argumentative. But she feels she can't leave Mom with the impression she's challenging her beliefs. She shifts in her chair before saying weakly: "I'm glad you feel God is on your side. You surprised me. I just wanted to make sure you're all right."

"With God on my side, how could I not be all right?"

The younger daughter nods but feels confused, her image of her mother suddenly shaken. At the same time, she experiences stirrings of something like envy. To feel such certainty, to know your prayers have been heard—it seems to her an incalculable gift, nearly incredible.

Even for people who wear their spirituality like a favorite sweater—warm, comfortable, and comforting—serious illness's chilling impact can make them feel as vulnerable as if they were stripped to the bone. Crises of faith—based on the conviction that disease is an unjust reward for the strivings of "good" people—are common. Crises of conscience—based on people's tendencies to blame themselves if they become ill, as if they're being punished for some transgression—occur even more frequently. It's not surprising, then, that from the Bible's Book of Job onward, religious thinkers have struggled to find some way to reconcile the pursuit of the moral life with the reality of human suffering.

Take several popular examples from our own times. In the classic book *When Bad Things Happen to Good People*, Rabbi Harold Kushner, reflecting on the death of his own 14-year-old son from a genetic malady, addressed these struggles directly. After exploring and then rejecting the idea that anything he or his son did could possibly have justified the advent of the son's illness, he concluded God must not be in full control of all that happens to us. Instead, he conceptualized God as a Supreme Being who has set the framework for existence but still battles against chaos in the universe—just as humans do. Rather than turning against God in anger, he recommended that suffering people ally with Him to rout out evils, such as illness.

More recently, Rabbi David Wolpe, writing in his best-seller *Making Loss Matter: Creating Meaning in Difficult Times*, focused not on why we sometimes suffer but on what we should do about it. He saw crises, such as serious illnesses, as opportunities for people to explore questions of their faith more deeply and to face the prospect of death more squarely—the better to learn and grow. He saw our capacity to derive meaning, including spiritual insights, out of even the most catastrophic medical event as the essential element of being human.

Pastor Rick Warren's blockbuster *The Purpose-Driven Life* (as well as the many similar titles it has spawned) approached questions of faith and suffering more indirectly. For Warren, discovering a sense of purpose shouldn't be the goal of any individual because each of us was brought into this world to be God's purpose. The true meaning of our lives is the significance with which God imbues us. For these purposes and meanings to be revealed to us, he believes we need only consult our "owner's manual," better known as the Bible. By placing our trust in God's plan, we can better accept the occurrence of untoward events, including disease and disability, because only He fully knows our ultimate purpose.

There are marked differences among these examples, particularly in the degrees to which they emphasize humans' capacity for adaptation or God's power to direct us. But there are similarities as well. Each author views anger at God in the midst of a medical crisis as counterproductive. Each sees such crises as times for strengthening faithful belief, not jettisoning it. Each ties belief to actions, such as prayer, rituals, and Bible study, and to a re-visioning of the world, either through spiritual revelation or by reawakening to the possibilities of our lives and of the finite moments on earth we're each granted.

These are the basic elements of a plan for you to sustain your spirit through a loved one's medical ordeal: Join with God to fight the disease; avoid making continued belief contingent on the outcome of your loved one's illness; and use the crisis as an opportunity for reflection, revelation, and transformation. There are as many ways to put these elements into practice as there are caregivers, with their own distinct beliefs, traditions, and predilections. Here are some suggestions I've seen prove helpful to hundreds of caregivers whose faith has been challenged:

• *When in doubt, seek religious counsel.* Paradoxically, the times many people seem least likely to seek out the guidance of a minister, priest, or rabbi is when their faith is shakiest or they're most riled at God. It's as if they fear their religious counselor will react to their discomfiture with umbrage, not understanding. (These concerns are most pronounced when they've had little previous contact or familiarity with the counselor.) But no spiritual guides worth their cloth are satisfied by preaching only to the choir. Their roles are to listen, sympathize, clarify doctrine, and mitigate doubts, not rake over doubters. Even if they aren't fully successful in these goals, their willingness to enter into ongoing dialogue with family members about these issues can do wonders for assuaging guilt that having doubts at all makes you unworthy of caring. Such dialogues aren't guaranteed, of course, to result in perfect resolution of all conflicted feelings or the dissipation of all confusion and anger. But they're a way for you to remain connected to your faith, if only by questioning it. With that connection intact, you retain much greater potential for finding a way to draw on the sustenance spirituality can offer than if you break all religious ties and opt for being alienated and aloof.

• *When feeling alone with illness, seek fellowship.* As we discussed in Chapter 3, seeking support is crucial for avoiding the enervating isolation of long-term caregiving. Before there were disease-specific support groups or national organizations advocating for caregivers' rights, there were local repositories of kindness called churches, mosques, and synagogues for caregivers to depend on. Some of the support these religious institutions provide is of the "covered casserole" variety—free meals, transportation, and other logistical assistance for families in need. As vital as this hands-on help is to keeping caregivers going, of even greater import is the sense of fellowship religious institutions can promote. Praying elbow-to-elbow with kindred spirits makes all prayers seem to ring louder, truer, and more powerfully. Kneeling together and rising in unison gives all congregants a greater sense of belonging. What's more, the church community generally defines a group bond of mutuality. When one community member is in need, others step forward. When those others fall on hard times, the ones who previously received now give aid. Those who need help are relieved of shame because they know in time they'll be called on to give back. Those who give help feel no burden because they know the day may come when they'll receive. No one is entirely alone with any travail. The sick and well are fellows beneath the same vaulted roof.

An interesting question concerning religious fellowship is whether the prayers of congregants foster the healing of seriously ill individuals. The very idea of research on this topic is controversial. Regardless of how fervently some people hold that prayer helps, many social scientists argue that this contention is a matter of faith and therefore not an appropriate subject for scientific study at all. Others who have gone ahead with such research have produced mixed results, with a few small studies finding that prayers do positively affect the outcome of disease while other projects have uncovered no discernible impact. What's more likely to be agreed on by all parties is that being publicly remembered by a spiritual community, if only through inclusion on a prayer list, can help make the ill and their caregivers feel less alone.

> Crisis raises hopes, beliefs, and superstitions that you may think your relatives never would have entertained in the past. If your ill loved one or another family member professes to have received some sign from a higher power or wants to take some preventive action that seems illogical but innocuous, expressing satisfaction that the person has found solace at such a difficult time acknowledges your relative's need to make some sense of the unthinkable.

• *When belief falters, bolster action.* Generally speaking, in Western religions congregants take up religious practices after they've established a belief in the precepts on which those practices are based. This isn't true in many Eastern traditions, in which belief not only doesn't precede action but may not be necessary at all for the participant to undertake a spiritual discipline. For example, in Japan many people take up Buddhism-influenced practices, such as ikebana (flower arranging) or kendo (swordsmanship), as explicit means of developing kokoro (spirit or heart) without subscribing to particular Buddhist beliefs about, say, the nature of reality or reincarnation. Studying these disciplines in the absence of religious beliefs doesn't make them any less effective for facilitating a meditative state of peacefulness and inner harmony. It's the experience of that beatific state that may then lead them to embrace certain beliefs about God and existence.

What this may say of pertinence to you if you're feeling angry is that if your beliefs falter, your actions must not. Staying the course of religious practice may ultimately lead you back to firmer grounding in faith. Or it may lead you to new spiritual byways with different but no less meaningful understandings of God. An example of this is when Rabbi Kushner, buffeted by his son's illness and death, eventually concluded that God must not control everything; this enabled him to retain his belief in the Lord's beneficence and justice.

Or consider the action of saying grace before meals. A disgruntled relative, soured by a loved one's steady slide, may resent the obligation of thanking a Savior who has seemingly ignored the family's prayers for restored health. But if he continues to say grace despite his sense of betrayal, he may find that, rather than ruminating about his disappointment with God, the prayer allows him a few moments of reflection on the goodness of his food. This contemplative stance will promote a greater awareness of his meal than he might ordinarily have. This greater awareness will lead him to relish with heightened intensity the miracle of nourishment—its tastes, textures, and variety. For some, this in and of itself will constitute a spiritual moment for which thanks will be given readily. For others, this moment of increased awareness may lead back to an appreciation for a God who would provide us with enjoyment of our delectable and life-sustaining repasts.

Another reason for bolstering religious practice falls into the category of "hedging your bets." None of us can be sure of the exact meanings of the adversities we face. Has God abandoned us, or is He just testing us à la Job? Is a dire medical outcome an eye-for-an-eye curse or celestial wisdom based on considerations we can't grasp? There's an old saying that when God closes a door He opens a window. Many of us who are angry at God, dubious of His purposes, or doubtful He even exists will say a prayer anyway—just in case. Better times may be around the next bend; we don't want to blow it with churlishness. We act because we don't really want to turn our backs. We act for the chance for ourselves and our loved ones to return to good stead, receive blessings anew, and glean insights we can't yet imagine.

Diverse religious thinkers and writers today agree on certain ways to make spirituality a blessing during medical crises and caregiving: Instead of being angry at God or making your faith contingent on your loved one's survival, join with God in fighting the illness; instead of giving up on religion when your beliefs falter, continue to follow some spiritual practice because it may lead you back to faith; instead of regarding the ordeal as only a loss, use it as an opportunity for spiritual growth.

Late morning on a cool, cloudy Sunday, the younger daughter dresses for church grudgingly. The mother had asked her, her sister, and their two husbands to attend a special healing service, and she didn't dare object for fear of the self-recriminations she'd experience if Mom died soon. But she's still brushing the lint off of her dress and combing her hair when her husband honks from the car for her to come out. She tramps down the stairs and puts on her coat with deliberation. It's not that she particularly wants to be late, but she feels a heaviness slowing her down. She isn't sure if it's resentment or obstinacy or a growing sadness that makes her balk and tarry. Slamming the front door shut behind her, she sways momentarily on the doormat, purposelessly studying the ornamental shrubs that line the driveway, before finally heading over to the passenger's side of the car.

Driving into the city, she's surprised her husband isn't grousing about having to go to church because it's an outing he usually resists like a dental appointment. If anything, he seems calmer than usual behind the wheel. It irks her, actually, making her feel all the guiltier for her reluctance. She has nothing against healing services. During her lifetime, she has been to several, for her grandparents and father, and found them to be touching family gatherings but not magical cure-alls. It bothers her that her mother seems to be placing so much hope in this one. The younger daughter stays quiet for most of the ride, glumly staring out the window while her husband keeps jabbing the preset buttons on the radio.

At the service, Mother is dressed in a very proper white skirt and blouse whose once bright fabric is now dulled with age. She looks thin and physically frail but sits erect in a second-row pew with eyes fixed on the minister at the lectern. The older daughter and her husband sit closely on either side of her. The younger daughter and her husband slide in next to them. Immediately the younger daughter feels distant from Mom and out of place. As her eyes become used to the dim light, though, she's reminded once again of how familiar these surroundings are. There's the stage where she was confirmed many years ago. There's the aisle down which her father walked her at her wedding. She looks around at the three dozen congregants scattered among the pews and recognizes none at first; it's been a long time since she came here regularly. But then her husband nudges her to look toward the back of the hall. Turning around, she sees an old female neighbor, now aged, with a daughter who was in her sister's and husband's class at school. What look like four adult grandchildren and their spouses and kids sit just behind them. The old woman, like the younger daughter's mother, appears careworn but alert. The younger daughter gives a faint wave, then pulls her arm down because she's unsure whether they'll recognize her after so many years. But the effect of simply seeing them has heartened her. It gives her a feeling she's come home to a place of old acquaintances coping with common concerns by employing common rituals. Looking around the church again, she sees other multigenerational clusters that could be her family rallying together to make a last stand against disease. She settles back against the pew's velvet cushion, feeling more relaxed and assured that she belongs here.

The minister is a stooped older man who, though not at this church when the younger daughter was growing up, has impressed her as a mild and caring person the few times she has met him over the past few years. The service he leads today is sober in tone but has a few light touches. There are traditional prayers and hymns but also poems—one by Rilke, another by the Canadian writer Margaret Atwood—as well as a rendition of a 1970s pop song "Morning Has Broken." The message is consistent: Have hope. Live each day. Embrace God. Toward the end, he invites up to the stage all the congregants seeking healing, to give each of them special blessings while placing his right hand on their shoulder or forehead. When mother goes onstage (with the help of the older daughter's husband), her eyes are wide, her expression serious. As the minister blesses her, she looks deeply moved.

After the service, they go down to the basement reception area for coffee and dessert. As they stand around the serving table, Mother is smiling. "When he touched my forehead," she says, "I had a feeling inside me that was different from before." Her older daughter and the two husbands listen to her, nodding. The younger daughter wants to support what she's saying, too, but feels herself recoiling a little because her mother seems so changed. She forces herself to say "Great, Mom" before drifting over to the pound cake. She thinks to herself there's nothing she would like more than for the touch of the minister's hand to eradicate mother's cancer. If only there is a God and He listens, it would be just. But, she reminds herself, the world doesn't revolve on "if only." Reaching for a piece of cake, she sighs, thinking at least her mother feels comforted.

To her surprise, the minister is suddenly standing beside her and strikes up a conversation. "Nice to see you again," he says warmly.

"Nice to see you, too," she replies. "I thought it was a very nice service."

"I'm glad you enjoyed it," he says. Then, without pausing, he adds, "Your sister has been telling me you've been struggling a bit."

"Oh?"

"I don't mean to put you on the spot," he continues, "but would you like to meet with me sometime soon to talk?"

The younger daughter is taken aback. The idea of airing her doubts about God terrifies her. Without meaning to be rude, she wheels around, seeking her sister, but sees that her sibling is across the room with her husband and Mom and isn't looking in her direction. The younger daughter's husband, however, is standing right in back of her. He must have heard the minister's offer, because he's nodding.

"These are hard times your family is going through," the minister says patiently. "Sometimes talking helps find a way to go on with your head higher."

"Okay, I'll call you," the younger daughter replies in a neutral voice.

"Good," he says. "I'll look forward to hearing from you." He sidles past her and joins another group of family members.

The younger daughter turns around again and looks at her husband. Before he can say anything, she says quietly, "Don't worry. I will."

Finding ways of sustaining your spiritual connections is invaluable for facing illness and uncertainty. It can become a bulwark for families through all rough stretches. When circumstances worsen despite prayers and blessings, however, families need all means for standing together against the onslaught of grief. In the next chapter, we'll examine possibilities for helping loved ones comfort one another and look toward the future without bitterness or strife.

Devout Acceptance or Passive Indifference?

Q: *My siblings and I want my mother to aggressively treat her cancer, but she's adopted what seems like passive indifference toward her disease. It's almost as though she's given up. "It's in God's hands," she keeps telling us. I know religious faith can help some people prolong their lives, but in my mother's case we fear her faith may actually shorten hers. What can and should we do?*

A: There's a very wide spectrum of religious beliefs about the ways patients should approach their medical treatments. At one end are extremely pious people, supported in their approaches by certain denominations, who eschew all treatment because they believe God will either heal them or not. At the other end are devout worshippers, equally supported by their creeds, who never refuse any treatment option because they believe God wants them to try to preserve life at every turn. In between these two poles are myriad possibilities based on a variety of beliefs—accepting some treatments but not others; pursuing treatment to a certain point and then refusing more; always pairing medical interventions with prayer or seeing prayer as wholly separate from pills and surgeries. In my opinion, these matters hinge on two key questions: Do you regard modern medicine as part and parcel of God's work (in which doctors and nurses are His hands on earth) or as the epitome of arrogant, technological secularism, antithetical to the primacy of belief in the Almighty? Do you believe God wants you to trust in the fate He's devised for you or use the judgment with which He has endowed you to try to save yourself? These are complex questions for which different individuals will arrive at divergent answers. One person's religiosity may be another's "passive indifference"; one's embrace of "aggressive" treatments may be another's disregard for God's will.

There seems like no more crucial time to have a discussion with your mother about her religious beliefs than during this high-stakes medical crisis. Before you and your siblings present your own spiritual views, though, you must demonstrate understanding of and respect for hers. Being respectful doesn't require you to agree with her; you can gently challenge facets of what she believes.

I'd start by inquiring about what she means when she says "It's in God's hands." Is she saying there's nothing she can do to alter what God has predetermined? If so, I'd counter with the suggestion that God might want her to fight the good fight by choosing treatment. Does working with her doctors mean to her she'd be working against God? I'd respond that you don't understand why she sees the two as virtual adversaries.

If respectful debate leaves her unmoved, ask her whether she'd be willing to attend a family meeting with her pastor or other religious leader. Such a meeting could achieve several aims: Your mother may receive clarification of religious doctrine that may permit her to accept treatment. It may offer her religious permission or dispensation to take medicine. You may be accorded a forum for expounding your own religious beliefs to help convince her to work with her doctors. On the other hand, a pastor might also work to help you and your siblings better understand your mother's deeply held convictions—even if declining treatment will probably result in her demise.

This last possibility would be very hard to accept. Not only might it offend your own religious beliefs, but it would likely devastate you and your siblings emotionally. And yet I doubt you'd deprive your mother of living out her life on her own terms. You'd wish the same for yourself from your children or any other family member. As she faces her battle with cancer in the manner she believes is best, she will need her family's embrace in addition to God's hands.

Finding Faith in the Wake of Anger

Q: *Since her mother died of cancer 3 years ago right before she gave birth to our first child, my wife has been very angry at God. She refuses to go to church or say prayers because they didn't help save her mother. I know my wife has had a strong faith that has given her a lot of strength during her life. I want her to be able to get over her anger and start to heal so she can lean on God again. I still do. How can I help her?*

A: Many people's sense of faith is tied to a conception of justice. They believe if they are moral and observant, they and their families will be divinely rewarded for their good deeds. When just rewards are not forthcoming, they are faced with a dilemma. On the one hand, they can conclude they weren't good enough and are consequently being punished. This is finger-pointing of the sort that decimates self-regard. On the other hand, they can question God's fairness or even His existence. This is pointing the finger outward in a way that ravages faith. It's not uncommon for this latter group to then refrain from going to church. Some people make this decision because they're too angry to enter a house of worship. Others see no point in attending services unless justice is done and their loved one is returned to them. Given the unlikelihood of this occurring, many never find their way back.

What path is there for you to help your wife return to faith? The key is encouraging her to reexamine her notions of God and justice. There are many questions she'd likely confront: Can there be a just God who allows people to suffer? If she can believe there's a larger plan we can't grasp in which individual suffering has significance, the answer can be yes. Are prayers heard if they're not answered? She'd have to consider whether her prayers really went unanswered or instead received responses she's still struggling to understand. Is your mother-in-law truly in a better place? If she reflects on the pain and debilitation her cancer was causing her mother and the additional agony she would have had to face, she may yet come to agree. You may want to converse with her about these difficult questions yourself. But it's also advisable to bring in a religious leader or teacher, if she'll abide one, to help frame these discussions for her.

While engaged in this soul searching, there are two questions concerning grief she also should address: Is holding on to anger at God preventing her from fully mourning her mother's death? If so, she may be inadvertently prolonging her own grieving process, leading her to suffer what psychologists call "complicated bereavement." This condition occurs when the normal grieving process of experiencing sadness and anger and then eventually recovering seems stuck. It's often associated with the development of major depression. That leads to the second question for her to consider: Have her many losses—including those of her mother, sense of universal justice, and grounding in faith—caused her to become depressed? If so, then it's possible her persistent anger at God is a manifestation of that depressed state. Counseling or antidepressant medication may decrease her depression and consequently lessen her anger at God. This may allow her once again to draw on her spirituality to find some semblance of peace about her mother's death.

Alternate Paths in the Search for a Cure

Q: *My ill mother has been influenced by a friend to pursue unorthodox alternative treatments and reject traditional medical treatments for her cancer. I feel it's a waste of time at best and dangerous at worst. How can I support her search for recovery but still make sure she isn't deluding herself or ignoring sound medical advice in favor of dubious practices?*

A: When "alternative medicine" first became popular in the United States about 10 years ago, it was seen as exactly that—an alternative to traditional technology-driven biomedicine, using "natural" remedies, such as ginseng, ginkgo biloba, and St. John's wort, and ancient practices such as acupuncture, as well as promoting spiritual beliefs to achieve greater health. However, an evolution in nomenclature and philosophy has occurred since then. Alternative medicine became "complementary medicine," an approach that saw the use of natural remedies as not an alternative but a complement to pharmaceuticals. More recently, complementary medicine has evolved further into "integrative medicine"—the natural and biomedical used seamlessly in close conjunction. There are still practitioners who emphasize the "instead of" or "alternative" approach. But especially in the field of cancer care—in which many hospital-based cancer centers now have integrative medicine programs, oncologists have greater familiarity with the use of natural remedies, and the remedies themselves have been better researched—patients' interest in nontraditional healthcare is generally welcomed.

Viewed within this historical context, your mother's decision to withdraw from traditional medical treatment is baffling and concerning. I believe it's better for her to entertain the use of natural remedies in consultation with her oncologist, who can at least guide her to those herbs and compounds with the best track records and research backing. She should continue talking with her oncologist, I'd contend, even if she decides to eliminate chemotherapy or radiation treatments from her health regimen. Unfortunately, there are many nontraditional practitioners hawking their unorthodox wares who prey on the fears of desperate people, especially end-stage cancer patients. It would be dismaying if your mother, once she turns her back on traditional oncology, were taken advantage of by these hucksters.

So how should you approach your mom? As always, family therapist Salvador Minuchin's famous saying "Join before confronting" is excellent advice. I recommend you gently ask her about her thoughts regarding her health and treatments. Before offering your own opinions, make sure she feels you've heard and understood her. Laud her for reaching out for any and all possibilities to beat her cancer because she loves life so much. But then carefully state your concerns. Tell her you love her and are afraid that the effect of her treatment decisions is going to shorten her life, not prolong it. Describe the integrative medicine approach as one that's inclusive enough to employ both traditional and unorthodox treatments. Ask her to at least consider sharing her thoughts with her oncologist and primary-care doctor. Tell her you'll support her as well as you can, regardless of which treatments she chooses.

In the end, as you know, the decision is hers; you should honor it as such. At least by raising the issue with her you'll have the satisfaction of having voiced your opinion about how she should proceed. More important, you'll have had the kind of lovingly broached "important talk" with her that will bring you closer together at a time of medical threat.

CHAPTER NINE

———————⌣———————

Last Days

Two weeks after starting her new chemotherapy, the mother awakens one morning to find her pillow covered with clumps of her own silvery hair. She'd been warned by her oncologist this might happen when he offered her the more aggressive treatment. But she had quickly agreed to it anyway because nothing else had worked. Today, though, she's aghast. Her hair was not thick to begin with, made thin and brittle by old age. Now, with wispy patches already appearing across her scalp in various spots, she looks and feels suddenly 20 years older. When her older daughter comes up to her room to check on her, the mother holds the pillow across the top of her head in embarrassment and requests some privacy. When her daughter chides her for being vain, Mother glares at her until the older daughter feels uncomfortable enough to retreat from the room.

In the mother's mind, vanity is the last sin of which she's guilty. She has never considered herself pretty, let alone a beauty. To the contrary, she knows that, on the most rouged-and-sequined, glamorously bedecked day of her life, she looked youthful but pleasantly plain. But now, after 2 weeks of every-other-day, 2-hour-long toxic infusions, watching her hair falling out—like observing cracked leaves showering down on a windy November day—has stripped her of the self-assurance of being familiar to herself. What she wants is the simple comfort of being able to recognize her puckered, silver-haired face in the mirror the one or two times a day she can actually bear looking. Instead, all she sees is cancer's ghoulish visage. Through the long course of an illness that has made her devitalized and dispirited, this seems the cruelest blow—that she herself would be transformed into a vision of disease, no longer looking so much like stalwart Mom as like the typical cancer patient.

The mother knows if she were to share these thoughts with her daughters, they'd hasten to convince her she is being too hard on herself. They'd tell her losing her hair hasn't caused her to stop being who she is. They'd probably also offer to get her a wig, as the nurses at the cancer center had suggested. But, for this mother, wearing some funny-looking hairpiece that resembles dyed straw or steel wool would only be adding another indignity for her to put up with. After fatigue and pain, intermittent nausea and (since starting the new chemo) profuse diarrhea, the loss of her apartment and the increased dependence on her daughters, the deterioration of her life enjoyment and the erosion of hope, she's unsure how many more indignities she can take.

As she throws another handful of her hair into the wastebasket and rolls over on her side, she muses to herself she knows better than to say things can't get much worse. They always can and frequently do. What devastation will be visited upon her next—locusts, vermin, or boils? The thought creeps into her consciousness that it may be better for the cancer to take her than for her to lose herself under an increasing barrage of indignities. Then she tries pushing that thought away as she rolls over onto her other side, noticing as she does more silver strands clinging to the front of her pajamas. She suppresses a sudden groan and then lies stiffly, hugging herself across her chest.

Later that day, Mother wears a blue-and-white silk kerchief over her hair when her daughters drive her over to the hospital for an appointment with her internist. She has seen him rarely in the past year since her initial diagnosis, when he turned her over to the oncologist's care. It alarmed her last week when she received a call from his receptionist asking her to come in for a complete physical exam. In the elevator up to the office today, she tugs at the edges of her kerchief, making sure it covers her scalp, fretting about the real purpose for which he wants to see her.

The internist, late as always, comes bounding into the exam room with his usual harried look. After a round of hand shaking and a gushy "great to see you," he explains to the mother he wants to thoroughly examine her to monitor how she's been holding up through the new chemo. He also wants to judge whether she could withstand radiation therapy after the chemo is done. "Radiation therapy?" the older daughter questions loudly.

"Oh, yes," says the internist. "When ovarian cancer has spread, it's one means we have of targeting metastases and prolonging the patient's life. I'm sure your oncologist must have explained it."

"He didn't," the older daughter shoots back.

The internist pauses and then says, "Well, I'm sure he was intending to soon."

The older daughter continues on the offensive. "Mom won't be able to handle radiation," she argues.

The internist pauses again. "I understand you're concerned," he says. "I promise you we'll take all care possible. Why don't you two excuse your mother and me now so I can get a clear idea of what she'll be able to tolerate?"

The daughters glance at each other and then get up and shuffle out to the waiting room. Sitting still on the exam table, the mother watches the internist with trepidation as he pushes aside boxes of rubber gloves and tongue depressors on the counter while hunting for his stethoscope. She actually wasn't surprised by the news about the radiation therapy. To turn this battle around, she assumed she'd need not only more powerful but more numerous weapons. But she has a suspicion there's yet another bomb the internist is going to drop today. Placing the bell of the stethoscope on her back and asking her to breathe deeply, he makes pleasant chitchat, saying at one point, "Your daughters are really caring," and at another, "This kerchief is pretty," before pronouncing that "Even though you have metastases, your lungs sound relatively clear and your heart is strong." Checking her reflexes with a small rubber mallet, he says in the same upbeat tone, "Good, good. You're holding up pretty well." When he helps her carefully get down off the exam table to take a seat next to the desk, he adds, "I wish most of my older patients had your fortitude. I believe you should be able to handle any new cancer treatments your oncologist has in mind."

He sits down on the blue swiveling stool and immediately begins thumbing through the many pages in her thick chart as if looking for something. The mother sits and waits for whatever he's about to say. "There are a couple of things we should discuss," he says after a few seconds. "I notice you have no living will. You know, it's a document to communicate your wishes for care in the event you're unable to speak for yourself at the time. I generally like to ask all my patients to fill one out at some point. I don't know how I missed asking you before."

Mother says nothing but thinks, He is preparing me for dying.

As if reading her mind, the internist quickly goes on, "I'm not bringing this up now because I think your treatment isn't going to go well. I have every confidence things will work out fine. But this is just a precaution." Seeing the grave look on her face, he adds, "I have a living will as well. Everyone should have one."

"If you think I should, then I'll fill one out," the mother says finally without enthusiasm. He gives her a gentle tap on her knee, then pulls a three-page form out of the desk drawer and hands it to her, saying, "I'll look forward to going over this with you when you're ready."

He then rolls his chair a little closer to her and leans forward as if speaking confidentially. "Before bringing your daughters back in," he says quietly, "there was one other thing. I referred you to your oncologist because I know he's highly competent. But I want you to know that oncologists in general are a very optimistic breed; they have to be to do the work they do. As long as you're willing to keep fighting, he'll come up with new treatments and options. If you ever want to stop treatment, you'll have to tell your oncologist directly. Otherwise, he'll just keep pushing new ideas to try."

He pauses to let Mother take this in and respond, but she's befuddled. Why is he saying this if he's so confident things will be fine? she wonders. But before she can formulate this thought into a courteous question, he hops up suddenly and leaves the room to bring in her daughters. When they return, he's back to chatting pleasantly. The daughters trail behind him with wary looks and take the seats next to their mother. As the older one notices the living will form in Mom's lap, her eyes widen. "Considering what your mother has been through," the internist says, "she's doing reasonably well and should hold up during her treatments. Of course, I'll monitor her regularly as she goes through this."

"What more will she be going through?" the older daughter asks sharply.

"I don't want to talk out of turn," he replies. "It's really your oncologist who should be discussing this with you." Seeing the dissatisfaction on their faces, he adds, "You know about chemo. Radiation is likely. Other options exist."

As mother and daughters mull over his last cryptic statement, he hurries on. "Let's meet in a month," he says as he gets up and strides toward the door. Then, as he touches the knob, he adds, "Don't hesitate to call me if you have any questions." In a moment, they hear him offer a gushy greeting to his next patient in the exam room next door.

On the way home in the car, the older daughter is tense with frustration and hits her brake pedal too hard at the first red light. She's irritated with the oncologist for keeping them in the dark and annoyed at the internist for his caginess. She'll call the oncologist and maybe the internist, too, to confront them both. But she dares not complain about them now because her mother needs to have faith in them; otherwise, how can they possibly help her? Glancing at Mom in the rearview mirror, she notices she's still holding the living will form. "Why did he give that to you?" she asks.

"He said it's a precaution," the mother says without emotion while gazing out the passenger side window. "He wants to know my wishes just in case I won't be able to say them." The older daughter responds only by saying "Oh." She and her sister exchange fearful looks in the front seat.

When they get home, Mother tells them she's very tired. The younger daughter helps her upstairs while her sister puts on a kettle in the kitchen. When the younger daughter comes down, she can tell by her sister's flushed face that she's in a huff. "These doctors treat us like a bunch of idiots," she complains. "Why can't they tell us everything that's going to happen?"

The younger daughter nods, partly in agreement, partly to appease her. She was irritated today but not nearly so much. The older daughter continues heatedly, "And what's with the living will? You'd think they were counting her out already."

"I don't think that's really it," the younger daughter says gently. "It's just what doctors do nowadays. And wouldn't you want to know what Mom would want us to do if she passed into a coma or something?"

"First off," replies her older sister, "it's like tempting fate. Why plan for bad things happening? Why not keep your hopes up by thinking about the good?"

The younger sister frowns but says nothing.

"Second," the older daughter goes on, oblivious of her sister's downcast expression, "I think we know what Mom would want if anything did happen."

"And what would that be?" the younger daughter asks.

The older daughter pauses and then says with more pressure, "Well, I believe she'd want to keep fighting and have all possible medical care. Isn't that what you believe?"

"I don't really know," the younger daughter says quietly. "That's why it's important for us to ask her and help her fill out the living will. Maybe she'd want everything done. Maybe she'd want only certain types of care under certain conditions. Maybe she'd want to stop all care and then go to a hospice—you know, stay at home and just have comfort measures. I don't know."

The older daughter is appalled by this last suggestion. "Mother wouldn't want a hospice," she says in earnest. "Dad fought to the end. It's in Mom's nature to fight to the end. It would be against her religion to give up on the chance to live."

The younger daughter is doubtful of this last statement but doesn't want to argue. She merely says again, "I don't really know."

There is a tense silence between them for a moment. They can hear the mother coming out of the bathroom upstairs. "Why are we talking about this? Mom's going to be all right," the older daughter says emphatically. The younger daughter nods in agreement again but is still thinking to herself, Really, I don't know.

When a medical crisis passes from the initial emergency stage to a chronic phase, you and your family members have to make adjustments in the ways you live to provide care and support over a prolonged period of time. Likewise there are adjustments to be made when the slow progression of an illness reaches a point at which the long-dreaded end comes into sight. (Perhaps your loved one's doctor believes the patient has less than 6 months to live and is therefore now eligible for hospice services.) You then have to rid yourselves of the illusions that the patient's condition is stable and that caregiving routines will go on indefinitely as they have for months or years. Instead, you should begin planning for the work of facing your loved one's probable death.

The most important part of that work is communicating together about practical, legal, and emotional issues. The practical issues revolve around supporting the patient to an increased degree as she declines physically or cognitively. You'll have to deal with the logistics of, say, providing 24-hour supervision for the patient, at home or elsewhere, if she now requires it or altering the home environment to make one-floor living possible if the patient can no longer negotiate stairs. Other practical questions might include "Should Mom sell the family home now and move into an institution?" or "Should we hire around-the-clock help for her?" or "Should we put together a schedule so there's a family member with Mom every night?" Family caregivers sometimes agonize over the answers to these kinds of questions, because they entail greater sacrifice and burden. At other times, though, they avoid even thinking about them by denying the reality that the patient is failing. There's a magical quality to the reasoning behind this: If planning for the needs of the patient is tantamount to accepting the patient's increasing neediness, then not planning for those practical considerations reinforces the false but comforting impression the patient is medically stable.

Close relatives may be just as likely to avoid convening a family meeting to discuss the legal issues that come up during a loved one's decline. These legal issues often include:

- Asking the patient about her "code status." Does she want all possible care in the event of a medical emergency (e.g., breathing tubes, respirators, antibiotics, full cardiac care), only certain interventions, or none at all?
- Asking the patient to fill out a living will or to designate a power of attorney (a particular individual to make medical or financial decisions for her in the event she isn't competent to do so).
- Writing a last will and testament.
- Transferring title of the family home to one of the adult children as a means for the family to possibly keep the house should the patient need to go into a nursing home.

These matters again confront everyone with the unbearable prospect that the patient will continue deteriorating to her death. There's also often fear the patient will interpret efforts to devise new legal arrangements as attempts to usurp her decision-making powers. Adult children of failing parents are especially chary to take these steps, anxious they'll be judged harshly for presumptuously acting "as parents to my parent." Discussions about these legal matters usually take place more easily when broached by primary-care physicians or hospital social workers as a standard aspect of patient and family healthcare. But even with the professional encouragement they provide, many family members are reticent about actually taking legal action by hiring attorneys, consulting bank managers, signing documents, filing papers, and so on.

Failing to act legally, however, can have exceedingly unpleasant results. The patient's medical condition may progress so rapidly that she doesn't have the time to express her wishes about the lengths to which she wants physicians to go to prolong her life. Without a living will or power of attorney, you're left to guess about—or, as often as not, argue vociferously among yourselves over—what the patient would have chosen or who should rightfully make the decision for her. Or the patient may have some precipitous downturn that makes it suddenly impossible for her to stay in her own residence. In those instances, the family home may have to be sold and the patient's savings withdrawn to help pay for long-term skilled nursing home care. (Many families feel justified in divesting the patient of all assets years before the need for nursing home care might arise so that the patient will be eligible for Medicaid to pay for those services; other families have ethical qualms about "spending down" their loved one's assets just to get governmental help.)

If you can resist denying the patient's decline, repress superstitions that planning will hasten her demise, and restrain fears of usurping a parent's power, then even more crucial emotional challenges arise as part of the psychological preparation for an impending death. Key among them, in the last days of a long illness, is tempering anger. Relatives often unite behind anger that's directed at the disease, the doctors, or even God. But they can as easily turn furiously on one another. Patients may blame caregivers for not standing nobly by them. Caregivers may blame patients for not battling hard enough. To feel disappointment in these instances is understandable. Fighting the good fight, praying with all your might, can make eventual loss all the more heartbreaking. But playing the blame game afterward is, as the saying goes, just stirring the bitterness in one's own cup—and heaping the dregs in the cups of every other family member. Anger upon anguish inflames pain. It covers over grief and prevents necessary healing. When families should be working hard to accept a medical loss and move forward as a loving unit, it keeps them second-guessing about the tragedies of the past.

During the initial and chronic phases of the patient's illness, most families consider sadness anathema to the mission of saving their loved one's life. But even when the end stage is at hand and sadness seems appropriate, many eschew it as a whiny indulgence and a weak-kneed throwing-in of the towel. More so than anger, however, deeply felt grief is considered by most psychologists to be therapeutic for family members who allow themselves to feel it. Rather than sapping the *esprit de corps* that the family may have gained through coordinated caregiving, shared expressions of sadness toward the end of the patient's life can create a feeling of communion that touches all members. That sense of togetherness when confronted with a common loss can shore up individual relatives through their mourning. It also can provide unspoken reassurance that members are still united and strong. It's as if members are demonstrating to one another that, despite the impending death of a cherished loved one, their family will endure and continue to care for its own.

The capacity to face impending loss with sadness and unanimity paves the way for you and the rest of the family to approach other emotional tasks. It's not every family's style to have long, lingering talks together. The stereotypical scene, dramatized in romance novels and tear-jerker movies, of loved ones speaking in hushed tones around the patient's bedside occurs in only a small portion of all caregiving families. Yet, without many words or deathbed vigils, family members who grieve together can still honor and forgive one another. Honoring a failing loved one is a matter of acknowledging her importance by taking the time to be present in her hour of need. It's also accomplished by reminiscing about and celebrating all the loved one has embodied during her life. Forgiveness doesn't need to be prompted by a formal apology or conveyed by its acceptance but can be requested and given by a soft pat on the shoulder or nod of the head or warm glance, as if to say wordlessly, "Serious illness reminds us life is too short. Let's drop all grudges and make good use of the time we have left."

When a crisis turns the corner from chronic to terminal illness, the caregiving family has to meet two critical challenges that will keep the family together and dignify the fight it has been waging:

1. *Undertaking practical, legal, and financial planning* that may stir up superstitions about hastening the patient's demise by "jinxing" him, cause discomfort over usurping your loved one's decision-making power, and throw everyone into denial that the end is near.
2. *Rejecting anger* that will tear the family apart and *embracing sadness* as a natural therapeutic part of facing loss.

Even when you've made honest efforts to address practical, legal, and emotional issues at the end of a loved one's life, you aren't in control of all you're about to face. Illnesses wax and wane and then wax again; sometimes it's hard to tell when the end of the patient's life has actually been reached. Relatives react in predictable and completely unforeseen ways. But by setting aside worries about upsetting others to plan for the last days, you can do your utmost to prepare for a range of contingencies. Once emotionally prepared as well as possible, you can turn your attention to other family concerns besides illness—at least for a little while. But as with all best-laid plans, what's expected to occur and the realities that unfold are never quite the same. The hope is that painstaking preparations will provide some buffer for the impact of what's to come. The truth is that not all of the impact can be buffered.

As sick as she felt on the more powerful chemotherapy, the mother wishes she were back on it. The radiation therapy she's getting now—three-times-a-week blasts to the nodules in her lungs—is more punishing. The skin on her chest and breasts feels scorched, though no black marks show. Her whole body feels devoid of energy. When she lifts up her head, weighty as a boulder, to glance into the mirror now, she's stunned not only by her bare skull—wiped nearly clean by the chemo weeks before—but by the deep red furrows beneath her vacant eyes. Even her older daughter has stopped telling her she looks fine. Mother senses now that her determinedly optimistic older child seems to be struggling to contain her shock at her parent's appearance. The younger child, quicker to express gloominess, just bursts into tears whenever she visits.

She's been ignoring their shock and tears, still holding out for some sort of miracle. Her daily talks with God have gone beyond simple praying to humble imploring to more urgent pleading: Just make this radiation work, why don't you? In time, her oncologist will order a new set of CT scans and other studies to see how effective the treatments have been. What he'll be looking for on the gray-shaded radiographic images is shrinkage of the nodules, hopefully to the vanishing point. No one on her healthcare team has been telling her how probable that is. She assumes, therefore, the chances are small. If they're the only chances she's got, though, she'll take them with God's help—hairless head and discolored face included. For all this suffering to be worth it, she knows she needs to halt the progression of the cancer, at the least.

The blank living will form still rests atop a pile of old newspapers on the kitchen table where Mother tossed it the day she came home from her internist's office. The older daughter notices it each time she walks into the room but keeps quiet because her mother seems bent on ignoring it. Once when the younger daughter came by, she picked up the three-page form and looked imploringly at her sister but then placed it back down quickly when she saw her older sibling's reproachful look. While she believes more strongly than ever their mother should define her wishes on paper, the younger daughter is hesitant to make more waves at this time.

Things are too hard nowadays. Not only has Mother's physical condition deteriorated, but hauling her back and forth to the hospital for treatments and appointments has drained the two sisters. Circling the garage seeking rare parking spots, sitting forever in stuffy waiting rooms with tattered magazines, getting headaches from the fluorescent lights—the routine has become oppressive to them. Compounding this, after more than a year since Mom's cancer was diagnosed, the daughters' husbands and children are flagging in their energy and openly chafing at the increased sacrifices they're being called on to make. The younger sister's spouse has been complaining about how infrequently she cooks now. The older sister's husband, much to his wife's ire, has been dropping comments that Mother might be better off in the city nursing home. Even the granddaughters have been carping that their mothers never come to see their own grandchildren. They're reluctant to go over to the older sister's house with their kids now because they're afraid their grandmother's ghastly appearance will frighten their children. All this has created greater strain for the two sisters because they feel the insistent tug of their own families while experiencing the increasing pull of their mother's descent.

The three women emerging from the hospital elevator on their way to the oncologist's office several weeks later are a picture of fatigue and anxiety. The older daughter, with jutting jaw and eyes straight ahead, looks morose but tough. Her sister's face is washed out. Mother is slightly hunched over, and her eyes have the dull glaze of resignation with sporadic flickers of worry. The radiation therapy ended the week before, and she underwent the whole-body CT scans a few days later. Today's meeting is intended for them to get those test results and, in her mind, to learn her fate. In the car on the way over to the hospital, her daughters had tried to talk her out of seeing this meeting in such absolute terms. "The internist said there are other options," the older sister had argued. The mother had remained silent but had thought, My options are dwindling.

The oncologist sits behind the desk in his office with the same formal air as usual. He inquires about how Mother's feeling, but his questions strike the daughters as perfunctory—small talk preliminary to the main proceeding. When he goes on to ask in greater detail whether she's had any headaches or dizziness, the younger sister feels annoyed and yet wonders if he's getting at something. The oncologist then opens the chart and launches into a lengthy recap of the events leading up to the mother's diagnosis and the various treatments tried thus far. As he drones on, all three women suspect he's engaged in a stalling tactic. The mother feels herself bracing for bad news.

As the oncologist's story of the mother's bout with cancer inches forward in time, he finally reaches the present circumstances. "About the results of your recent CT scans," he says gravely, "I'm sure you've been anxious about them." He pauses, and the three women stare at him, waiting for him to stop the dramatic build-up and go on. The older sister says in a voice barely masking irritation, "Yes, we've been anxious. Please do tell us."

The oncologist flips through the chart again until he finds the radiologist's report and then says, "There are findings both good and bad. What we hoped to see is that the combination of the chemotherapy and radiation, or perhaps just the radiation alone, would shrink the lung tumors we were so worried about. That, in fact, has happened. The nodules haven't been completely eliminated but have been significantly reduced in size. By any measure, that's a very good sign of partial treatment success."

He pauses again. The mother worries about exactly what he means by "partial treatment success." Will she be only partially well? Or will the cancer only partially kill her? The older sister cuts in once more, asking, "And the bad findings?"

The oncologist hesitates for a beat and then continues in the same deadpan voice. "The radiologist and I aren't entirely sure of this yet," he says carefully, "but I'm afraid there are indications on the CT films the cancer may have spread further."

The three women momentarily stop breathing. "What? Where?" the older sister bursts out.

"I'm afraid it may have spread to your mother's brain," he says. The women all stare at him. As in an earlier meeting many months ago, Mother begins to well up.

The oncologist hands her a tissue and says, "Allow me to share some of my thinking with you. We need to do more testing before we can make any definitive conclusions. Metastases to the brain would be a serious development. But, as I said, not all of the news is bad. The fact that your cancer may have spread is likely an indication the two forms of chemotherapy we've used so far have not been especially effective. There are other, more powerful types of chemo we can use. But we also know that the radiation seemed to reduce the nodules in your lungs. There's a fair chance that radiation therapy, carefully directed, could help eliminate many of the cancer cells in your brain."

He looks at the faces of the mother and her two daughters and sees they are overwrought. "I've probably already given you too much information at one time," he says. "We should probably meet again soon to talk more after you've had time to absorb this. The next step is to do more testing."

The three women say nothing at first. Mother is still dabbing her eyes with the tissue. Then the younger sister asks quietly, "What would be the side effects of radiation on Mom's brain?"

"Well," says the oncologist, meticulously choosing his words, "there's always the possibility of increased fatigue, decreased intelligence, even changes in personality. But we have ways of reducing those risks by finely directing the therapy, implanting radioactive seeds, or possibly other options."

The mother thinks to herself that at every turn there always seem to be "other options." Each, of course, appears to have its noxious drawbacks. She recalls the internist's words that it would be up to her to decide when to tell the oncologist she'd had enough. "Thank you for taking the time to explain all this to us," the mother says graciously. "I'll certainly go for whatever tests you suggest." The oncologist fills out and then hands them prescription slips with instructions. When Mother rises unsteadily from her chair, each daughter jumps up to grab hold of one of her elbows. They then slowly depart the office silently.

They maintain the silence in the elevator back downstairs and during the long walk to the parking garage. As they shuffle along, the older sister sneaks glances at her mother to try to read not just her state of mind but the workings of her brain. Has cancer already affected Mom's thinking and personality? she wonders. She hadn't noticed that Mom has been more forgetful than before she became ill. But, for some time now, she's observed that Mom has lost much of her spunk and fire.

Is that a result of cancer-induced neurological damage or just difficulty coping? The older sister can't tell.

When the older sister unlocks the car doors, the younger sister suddenly breaks the silence. "Maybe we should go to another hospital for a second opinion?" she asks. The daughters look at their mother for a reply. She says slowly, "I'll consider it. I'm not against that idea, but I'm generally satisfied with the oncologist I have. I'm tired. I don't feel strongly about it either way." The three of them climb into the car, and Mother adds, "Well, let's go home and get that living will form in the kitchen. I suppose I'm now ready for it."

When a loved one dies suddenly from a heart attack or stroke, his relatives are often caught unaware and react with a slew of emotions we call a state of mourning. In her 1969 book *On Death and Dying*, the late Swiss psychiatrist Elisabeth Kübler-Ross described these reactions to death as an ongoing process or a series of stages over time that includes shock, anger, depression, and acceptance. Subsequent studies by other researchers have supported a range of expectable emotional reactions but not in a set sequence. Rather, different emotions are experienced at various times and in different orders, depending on the individual's idiosyncrasies, family traditions, and cultural backgrounds. Perhaps Kübler-Ross's greatest contribution to Americans' approach to death was in showing that it's all right to still be mourning the loss of a significant relative or friend long after the funeral is over, the condolence cards have been stacked in a drawer, and the deceased's clothes have been cleared from the closets. We aren't required to put our feelings of grief quickly aside and "get on with life." On the contrary, we're allowed to remember, cherish, and feel for as long as we need to.

Kübler-Ross, among many other mental health clinicians (including family therapists Evan Imber-Black and Janine Roberts, who have written extensively on the topic), advocated the use of rituals as a prime means for helping people deal with their grief. A ritual is a culturally or family-prescribed set of activities that allows individuals to express strong feelings through a structured activity and within the context of a supportive community. Common death rituals include funerals and memorial services, sitting shiva (for Jews) and attending viewings (for Catholics), planting trees, dedicating benches, scattering cremated ashes in places the deceased loved, and gathering together at bars, barbecues, and borough halls to swap favorite remembrances. At each of these events, family members can beat their breasts with sadness, tell raucous stories or ballyhoo the lessons learned from their loved one's life—all with the sanction of the group of fellow mourners present. The sense of togetherness engendered by such rituals boosts people's spirits at a time of loss while also implicitly providing assurance the family and community still survive and life for all involved continues forward.

There's another kind of grief that affects patients and family members dealing with chronic progressive illnesses, such as Alzheimer's dementia, severe coronary artery disease, and many types of cancer, which has been termed "anticipatory loss" by psychiatrist John Rolland. If the ultimate goal in dealing with bereavement is acceptance, then the goal of contending with anticipatory loss is continued emotional engagement. Knowing a loved one is likely to die soon often causes an upsurge of diverging feelings—sadness, worry, anger, relief, guilt. The intensity of these ambivalent emotions is uncomfortable to bear, leading many family members to distance themselves from the unfolding tragedy as a means of protecting themselves from their own strong reactions. Yet, as we discussed earlier, it's also a time when the patient's increasing needs create greater demands on family members to be in close proximity to provide help. As a consequence, a relative's need for greater distance and the patient's need for closer care can clash. This conflict may lead to one of several hurtful scenarios: The family member keeps away and the patient feels neglected; the family member provides the increased help mechanically and emotionlessly and the patient feels uncared for; or the family member provides the increased help in a heightened state of emotional tension and the patient feels resented.

To handle anticipatory loss without alienating the patient and consequently "losing" her any sooner than is necessary, you and your family members should consider taking several steps:

- Be aware that facing the reality of a loved one's impending death often spurs a nearly reflexive urge among family members to pull away.
- Minimize the impact of this urge on your actual behavior by enhancing your awareness of it but also by discussing it frankly with other family members (who, though chagrined, probably feel similarly), hospice workers, and other healthcare professionals.
- Don't share your intense feelings with the patient, even if she has long been your best friend and confidant. Enlisting her as your

supportive listener now may inhibit her from vocalizing all she is thinking and feeling when time is short.

- Balance conversations with other family members about ambivalence with planning sessions about how each will fairly do his part to comfort the patient until the end.
- Consider using hospice services months before the patient's death. Providing support with anticipatory grief is one of the primary roles of its grief counselors and chaplains.

If these steps are taken, anticipation of the patient's death will have served as preparation for and mitigation of later bereavement. You'll avoid the guilt that often arrives at the funeral about not having done enough (or, possibly, anything at all) for your loved one while she was alive. You'll also have sidestepped the resentment of other relatives by not letting them down at a time when all members are expected to contribute. The sadness you allow yourself to feel during the drawn-out time prior to your loved one's passing will lessen the shock of grief and shorten the period of deepest mourning when family life seems abjectly grim.

Skillful handling of anticipatory grief can keep you close to your loved one at a time when you may instinctively distance yourself to protect yourself from intolerable pain. It can also pave the way for more productive mourning and less guilt over whether you did enough while your relative was alive.

Mother had been so fearful of the radiation treatment to her brain that she'd expected immediate cataclysmic changes—a burning sensation inside her skull that would scorch her abilities to think and feel in the exact ways that make her who she is. But 3 weeks into the therapy, she considers the side effects thus far to have been relatively mild, including a warm itchiness at her right temple and a slight fuzziness to her thoughts. She believes the latter is as likely due to her stubborn fatigue as to any damaging radiation to her nerve cells or spreading cancer growth. Otherwise her days have been much the same as before—dragging up and down the stairs, frequent hospital runs, picked-over meals, hours stretched out on her bed. She's been feeling neither despondent nor hopeful lately but instead mostly numb, waiting for whatever is to come. This morning she's waiting for another brain scan and a reexamination by her oncologist to monitor the effectiveness of this latest medical intervention.

Soon she's sitting in the backseat of the car again with her daughters up front on the too-familiar route to the hospital. Soon after she's sitting again before the big desk in the physician's office, and he's looking like his starched, officious self. She's especially fuzzy now or maybe just particularly numb, and everything feels a little unreal to her, as if it were taking place in a TV melodrama about serious doctors and frightened patients. She can see by the tight expressions on her daughters' faces they're very anxious for the latest report, but she, perhaps self-protectively, can't feel any anxiety herself. When the oncologist frowns as he views the latest CT scans on the light box and says the brain metastases have not yet shrunk, she watches her daughters' postures slump but changes neither her own bland expression nor her rigid perch on the seat's edge. When she hears the oncologist go on to say they should go forward with an even stronger chemo—an experimental drug in trials at the major university medical center on the other side of the city—she finds herself nodding as if in agreement though she's unsure how she really feels. Later on, in the elevator back downstairs, the thought crosses her mind that she doesn't like the idea of an "experimental drug"; it sounds like she'll be some kind of guinea pig whose torment will help "science" or someone else but not her. But even this unpleasant notion flits through her mind lightly and is gone rapidly. After returning to her older daughter's house, she avoids her children's pained silence by excusing herself without explanation, lamely pushing her walker away from the kitchen table, and slowly climbing the stairs to her room.

Once there, she settles onto the bed and, as her head touches her flat pillow, begins to feel her emotions surfacing to her conscious awareness. She feels angry at first—at God, the doctors, her failing body—and her face suddenly hardens into a scowl. But just as quickly, her pursed lips start quivering and tears are streaming across her wrinkled cheeks. She sobs hard for nearly a minute, then her breathing relaxes though the tears continue to flow. After several more minutes, the jag has abated and she's sniffling but no longer crying. With pent-up emotions now relieved, she feels better and, for the first time today, can think clearly. She pushes herself awkwardly into a sitting position on the bed, takes a deep breath, and then stands up. As she glances around it occurs to her how strange life is, to find herself old and crying here amid the juvenile decor of her granddaughter's former room. She hobbles over to the window facing onto the front yard and looks out. There, again, is the shiny glint of the wet grass, though on a different patch of lawn than weeks before. She recalls with bitter irony that she once took it as a sign of better things to come.

Leaning heavily on the windowsill, she wonders if the brightness could be a sign of something else. As she scans the trim green yard, she notices the light reflecting from it is of varying intensities in different spots, depending on the amount of grass and moisture in any one area. It makes her think of the "brightness" or goodness in the world, more evident in some places and with some people, less apparent at other places and with other people. She thinks, too, of the bright and dim periods in her own life; seen as a whole like this variegated carpet of lawn, it would seem like a patchwork of swirling shades, depending on the angle and intensity of light. She tells herself, "I believe God is the light that reflects on my life. He's brightened some of my days to the point of glowing. He's darkened others to the point of gray despair. They're all part of the same whole, though." Still scanning the lawn, it seems to her at this moment like some beautifully verdant expanse. Still reflecting on her life, bright and dim, it strikes her it has been a mostly beautiful expanse as well.

The mother hesitates at the sill an instant longer, then shuffles back over to the bed and sits down. After thinking for a minute more, she begins to make her way downstairs. Hearing their mother slowly descending, the daughters pop out of the kitchen and look up at her on the staircase with questioning looks, surprised she has reappeared. They help her down the remaining steps and then escort her over to the kitchen table. The older daughter immediately puts on the kettle for tea. "There's something I'd like to discuss with you girls," the mother says. They glance at each other and then take the seats on either side of her.

"I know this has been an upsetting day for all of us," the mother says. "I'd like to spare us other meetings like that. On the whole, I think I've had a very good life. I really have no complaints."

The daughters wait for her to go on, but she just looks back and forth at them solemnly. They look at each other, confused. "What is it you're saying?" the younger daughter asks.

"I've had good and bad times in my life," Mother replies. "That's the way God has fashioned it. I can accept that."

"And?" asks the older daughter.

The mother responds, "And I don't want any more chemo or radiation. I'll let things take their course."

The daughters are motionless for a prolonged moment until the shrill whistle of the kettle prompts the older one to get up and turn off the burner. When she sits back down, she states bluntly to her mother, "You can't do that."

Her younger sister answers her quietly, "It's her choice. Yes, she can."

The older sister ignores her. She says to Mother, "This isn't you. You don't give up. This isn't what God would want."

The mother takes a long time to answer her before saying, "I've felt very close to God recently. I believe this may be what He wants. And I think it's what I want."

There's silence again. The older sister starts crying and says, "This is very hard for me."

The younger sister says, "This is hard for all of us. Don't make it any harder for Mom."

The older sister answers her angrily, "You've been nothing but gloom-and-doom from the beginning."

Her sister responds instantly, "That's not true or fair."

"Stop it," their mother says brusquely, the old matriarch yet. "Fighting isn't going to make it any better. I'm afraid you may have to lean on one another to deal with what's going to happen because of what I've decided."

The older sister starts crying harder. She mumbles through gritted teeth, "Excuse me," and gets up from the table. Her mother and younger sibling watch but don't try to stop her as she bolts from the room.

In the weeks that follow, the younger daughter can only describe her experience as a blur, like the trees and mile markers slipping past in the corner of her eye as her car hurtles toward her sister's house each morning. With Mother's decision to stop treatment, the clock on her life seems to have started running faster, and, as a consequence, all of reality seems sped up. The younger daughter feels harried and exhausted and a little out of control.

The follow-up meeting with the oncologist had gone reasonably well but had still been unsettling. When the mother had explained to him she was no longer interested in treatment, he'd visibly stiffened and then begun questioning her in detail about her judgment. But when it was apparent after 10 minutes that she wouldn't budge, he'd surrendered, smiling faintly and inviting her to see him again if she should change her mind. Mother had thanked him for all his efforts; so had the daughters. As they were heading out of his office, however, the oncologist's smile had sagged for an instant into a look of sadness. The expression had bothered the younger daughter, making her feel guilty for supporting her mother against his evident good intentions. She didn't want to fight against his desire to fight on; she really wanted to justify his hard work by finding some way to save her. His look had also added to her uncertainty about whether Mom's decision was truly the right one.

Since the initial uproar at the time of Mother's announcement, the younger daughter had observed her sister closely for signs of further outbursts. But in the ensuing days, the older sibling had regained her composure quickly and seemed all the surer about the proper course of action for Mother to take. Mother told the younger daughter that, during several late evenings, her sister had sat in the upstairs bedroom pleading with her to opt for any of the available cancer treatments. Contemplating this now as she exits the highway and decelerates quickly, the younger daughter is saddened by the image of that scene and yet impressed her mother has withstood her sister's pressure. But she's even more struck by the irony that Mother seems intent on maintaining control over her life by exercising her prerogative to quit fighting and die. The younger daughter feels greatly moved by this effort at self-determination. At the same time, when she imagines the fulminant cancer spreading through her mother's brain, lungs, and other internal organs, she can't help but feel literally nauseated.

Pulling into the driveway and letting herself into the house through the unlocked front door, the younger daughter finds her sister with hunched shoulders and a drowsy look sitting in her usual chair in the kitchen. The older daughter announces wearily, "Mom's still upstairs sleeping," without waiting for her sibling to ask. The younger daughter picks up the morning paper lying at the end of the counter and then sits down at the table. Neither talks very much; in fact, they haven't done so for weeks. In the slightly awkward silence between them, both harbor awareness of their difference of opinion about what Mother should do. Neither desires any conversation that might lead to an ugly argument. There's not much more to say anyway—only wait. The younger daughter runs her eyes over the front page's headlines disinterestedly. Her sister gets up suddenly and says, "I have to run some errands. I'll be back in a couple of hours." The younger daughter just nods and scans the paper again.

After the older daughter pulls the front door shut behind her, stillness comes over the house and makes the younger sister feel a little spooked. She tosses the paper aside and fusses about the kitchen, scrubbing the week's worth of tea-stained mugs in the sink. Without giving it much thought, she then finds herself tiptoeing up the stairs and cracking open the door to her mother's bedroom. The old woman is still sleeping on her side beneath the crocheted blanket, looking peaceful and vulnerable as a child but also sharp-boned and spindly as a crone. The younger daughter stares at her while thinking about how different this person seems than the vibrant mother she's always known. As if sensing her presence, the mother suddenly opens her eyes and struggles to sit up. "I'm sorry to wake you, Mom," the younger daughter says. But the old woman only looks around the room, seemingly confused. After a few moments, the younger daughter asks, "Are you okay, Mom?" Her mother nods, but her eyes are still unfocused. Finally, she asks in a hoarse voice, "Is it nighttime?"

"No, it's mid-morning," the younger daughter responds. Then, opening the blinds, she says, "Look," as streaming yellow beams immediately brighten the dim, stale room. At once, Mother lies flat on her back and covers her eyes with her forearm, saying, "I'm going to go . . . go . . . go . . . ."

"What, Mom?" the younger daughter asks. She knows that, because of the burgeoning cancer in her brain, her mother has begun to have trouble finding the right words when she speaks. "Going where, Mom?" asks the younger daughter again.

The old woman remains in the prone position and doesn't answer. The younger daughter asks again, "Going back to sleep?" The mother says, "Yes." The younger daughter then closes the blinds and scampers out of the room.

By the time she reaches the kitchen, the younger daughter is already crying. Seeing her mother losing the energy that made her feisty and the quick tongue that made her formidable is too much for the daughter to bear. She sits down heavily again at the table, thinking that, just as with her father, worse heartbreak is to come.

Two-and-a-half months later, the older daughter is in the kitchen griping on the phone to the hospice nurse. "But you said you'd be here by 10 o'clock," she fumes. "My mother has to be cleaned up and changed." In a moment, she puts the receiver down firmly. It's ridiculous, she thinks, that the nurse comes only once or twice a week and more absurd yet she's consistently a half-hour to 2 hours late. What good does it do her mother or herself to let some stranger into the house who's not even reliable? But the internist had suggested hospice, her younger sibling had insisted on it, and Mother had acquiesced. The best the older daughter could say for herself is she had gone along. She knows it was better than acceding to her husband's wish to have Mom spend her last days in a nursing home. But it galls her that, having been magnanimous in accepting a hospice plan she never would have chosen, she has wound up doing the bulk of her mother's care because the nurses, social workers, and aides are tardy and her sister recently has become scarce.

Before heading out of the kitchen, the older daughter picks up a plastic box of wipes and a container of talcum powder from the counter. The mother's now spending all of her time lying in an oversized hospital bed with smooth gray railings in the living room. Once the house's pristine showcase, the room now has the forest of IV poles and tubing, stacked metal basins, and scattering of white sheets, towels, and cotton dressings of a small surgical suite. Mother watches her daughter enter the room but says nothing. A TV set on a rolling tray at the foot of her bed is airing a morning talk show, but the sound has been muted. With a glance, the older daughter notes that her prone mother, with folds of loose skin beneath her neck contrasted by gaunt cheeks, has been losing weight. "How are you, Mom?" the older daughter asks. There's a pause and then the mother answers groggily, "All right." Her words come thickly because the morphine drops the hospice nurse instructed the daughters to give her for pain every few hours tend to sedate her into either a torpid haze or a stuporous sleep. "Do you want something to eat?" the daughter asks. Again the mother pauses before shaking her head no. A couple of weeks ago, the daughter would have taken it personally that Mother was rejecting the food she was offering. With the help of the educational materials provided by the hospice nurse, she now understands the drug also suppresses her appetite, not to mention constipating her whenever she does ingest something. There's no joy in eating—or anything else, it seems—for her mother anymore. It's very painful for the daughter to see, but she's learned to bear it by reminding herself that it's all part of Mom exercising her ultimate choice.

"There's no telling when the nurse is going to show up," the older daughter explains. "Let's change you now." An anxious look appears in Mother's eyes. Because her balance has become poor with her increasing brain dysfunction and weakness, it's too hard to get her to the bedside commode most of the time. As a consequence, she has taken to wearing disposable diapers during the last few weeks. Wearing the diapers hurts her pride; having her daughter change them humiliates her. As the older daughter pulls back her sheets and blanket, the mother braces herself as if for something painful. The older daughter notices, places her hand gently on Mother's shoulder, and says, "I know. It's okay." The mother relaxes a little, and the daughter goes about her business with wipes and powder. It hurts her, too, to see her mighty mother brought so low, but it has to be done. It's really no different, she reasons, than changing one of her grandbabies. Afterwards, when the daughter has put the sheet and blanket back on her, Mother says slowly with tear-filled eyes, "Thank you. I'll never forget you." The older daughter says matter-of-factly, "I know."

It's only when she heads into the kitchen to wash her hands that she allows tears to fill her own eyes. She's sad but also excruciatingly frustrated to be so helpless to save her mom. She looks at the clock and sighs, figuring the nurse who's coming to check on Mother's condition and replenish her morphine supply will probably be even later than she'd promised on the phone. And where is her younger sister? It's getting on toward noon, and there's been no word from her. The older daughter grabs the receiver and punches the speed dial. "So, where are you?" she asks as soon as the younger daughter picks up.

The younger daughter is immediately on the defensive. "I'll get there," she responds with annoyance. "I had to run some errands."

"I'm sure you did," the older daughter says archly. "But I don't mean just this morning. Where are you in general nowadays? Since you got us all involved with hospice, you just don't come around and help the way you did before."

The younger daughter's first impulse is to deny it. "That's neither true nor fair," she protests strenuously with her usual line. But when her older sibling doesn't respond at all, the silence works on the younger daughter's guilt. She realizes she's been increasingly reluctant to go over to her sister's house as their mother has declined. "Well, maybe I haven't come by as much," she says less gruffly, "but it's been hard for me to see Mom in the state she's in."

The older daughter answers in a calm voice without malice, "To quote you, 'It's been hard for all of us.'" The younger daughter says nothing. The older sibling then goes on: "I know you're more sensitive than I am. I don't want you to get depressed again. But Mom and I need your help. I don't think she has much time."

The younger daughter says with resignation, "Okay." She pauses and then adds sadly, "I can't explain how much I hate this. She doesn't deserve this; neither do we." The older daughter starts to answer, but the younger sibling cuts in and continues: "I know you know this. I appreciate your concern about me. I don't want you to have to do everything. See you in an hour—maybe two. I will try to be there more."

The older daughter just answers, "Fine."

A few weeks later, the hospice nurse informs them that Mother seems to be approaching her end. Her breathing is shallower, she's sleeping even more, and, when awake, her thoughts are increasingly confused. Some of this may be due to the higher dosages of morphine the daughters are administering because of their mother's mounting pain, but, as the nurse keeps emphasizing to them, a death with dignity shouldn't include agony. In light of the nurse's prediction, the daughters organize an around-the-clock vigil so that either one of them or their husbands or daughters are with Mother at all times. They pray that God forbid she die alone.

The woman in the hospital bed in the living room bears little resemblance to the once powerhouse matriarch of this family. She spends nearly all of her time lying in bed with her head up against one of the gray railings, mussing the strands of scraggly silver hair that have grown back since she stopped treatment. Her skin is pale and mottled, and spittle clings to the corners of her lips. The old house dress she wears is twisted about her body and widely stained. The younger daughter can't believe how shabby she looks. In her mind, her mother has already died. Why have they all worked so hard to caregive her, she wonders, if it comes down to nothing more than watching her suffer before dying? She feels cheated. Her older sister may feel the same way, but she continues to protect herself with busyness—rushing around, changing sheets, fixing meals for the other family members who have come, calling the hospice nurse with updates.

One day Mother is more alert than she has been in several weeks. Her pain seems diminished, and she requires less morphine. When the younger daughter arrives that morning, she finds her mother sitting upright in the raised hospital bed, sipping ice water from a straw the older daughter holds for her. The mother stops sipping when the younger daughter comes in and gives her a wan smile—the first in a long time. The younger daughter comes over to the bedside and takes her mother's hand. Mother squeezes it lightly and then looks at the older daughter and smiles at her as well. As the daughters watch their mother's face, she tries to speak but is too weak to make much sound. Instead, she mouths what clearly looks to the daughters like the phrases "Thank you" and "I love you." There are other things she mouths that they cannot quite make out. Later on, the younger daughter will come to believe that one of the phrases is "I'm going to join your dad."

It's the mother's last hurrah. That afternoon she drops into a deep sleep during which her breathing becomes slower and shallower. After a while, there's an alarming rasp to her breaths that's grating to the daughters' ears. When the older daughter calls the hospice nurse about it, the nurse tells her death is near. The daughters then get on their phones and call the family together. Both of their husbands rush there from work. Most of the granddaughters arrive, some with their spouses. They stand around the living room or wait in the kitchen. Because she's laboring to breathe, Mother's face looks strained as if she's suffering. It causes anguish for her family members to watch her. They want the reassurance to know she'll go peacefully. As the hospice nurse had instructed, the older daughter gives the mother more morphine drops through her parted lips to alleviate her agitation and keep her more comfortable as the pain increases. As evening wears on, something seems to be shifting. Her breaths are coming slower, and her facial muscles seem to have relaxed. At last, around 8 o'clock, Mother takes one deep breath and then lets it out slowly for what seems a long time. She doesn't breathe again after that. Her face looks impassive and smooth. The daughters and granddaughters cry. The older daughter's husband says the Lord's Prayer. While the older daughter goes to call the funeral director, the younger daughter puts up a large kettle of water for tea.

As they wait for the funeral director to come take Mother's body away, the two daughters sit quietly in the living room with her. After a year and a half of caregiving, the younger daughter feels relieved, saddened, exhausted, and numb. She chokes back fresh tears every few minutes. The older daughter has returned to a more stoic restraint. She gets up after a few minutes to brush Mother's wispy hair and to try to smooth out the remaining wrinkles from her brow. They can hear their daughters talking and even laughing in the kitchen. One is telling another, "Do you remember the time Grandma got mad at us and chewed us out in church?"

The funeral takes place in that church a few days later. The daughters and their families sit in the two front pews, but they have placed a large bouquet of flowers in a pew toward the back of the hall because that was where their parents would sit whenever they'd come here. Years before, Mother had requested that her service be exactly the same one—songs, psalms, and all—her husband had a decade ago. So, as the daughters sit through the hour-long proceedings, they feel sorrow over the loss of their mother but also renewed grief for their father. Yet, not all of their feelings are sad. Looking around, they each can see themselves walking down this church's aisle at their weddings and those of most of their children, too. There have been confirmations and baptisms here as well. The place seems to hold the joys and sorrows and sense of continuity for the whole family.

Later, at the large family cemetery plot, the younger daughter stares at the many headstones of mostly beloved deceased relatives and feels afraid. She leans over toward her sister at one point during the minister's oration and whispers solemnly, "Everyone in the family who was older than us is gone. We're next." Rather than eliciting her older sister's fear, her sibling immediately guffaws, cracking, "Good. I can use the rest." The younger daughter feels ridiculous in her anxiety and smiles. Later on, however, as the mother's casket is being lowered into the ground, it's the older daughter who leans toward her sibling to express some feeling of dread. "We're orphans now," she says. Though it also strikes the younger daughter as a little ridiculous for two adults in their fifties to think in those terms, she knows what her sister means. Mother is dead. They are alone with one another. The two sisters hold tightly onto each other and sob hard as their daughters and husbands crowd around to press close to them.

A Daughter Asks How Far She Should Look Down the Road Ahead

Q: *Our mother has had a progressive debilitating disease for 30 years. She now needs help from our father with everything, every day. Lately, I've found myself thinking more and more about the future and wondering how much more disabled she'll become. Will she end up completely immobile? How much will my father be able to handle? Dad will never agree to put Mom in a nursing home; he'll work himself to exhaustion instead. My two brothers don't like to think about such possibilities, but I think we have to in order to head off a crisis one day for her and him. How can I handle this?*

A: When a loved one starts down the path of a chronic, progressive illness, like Parkinson's disease, Alzheimer's dementia, or certain types of multiple sclerosis, most family members don't want to look too far down the road. Without some medical miracle to sidetrack the disease's course, the inevitable devastation at the end is too dispiriting to contemplate. Most patients and family members at the beginning or middle of the journey adopt a "one day at a time" philosophy, focusing on today's troubles to keep themselves from being daunted by tomorrow's more heart-wrenching catastrophes. Planning for future contingencies does require some familiarity with a map of the path ahead. But most people still choose to keep their eyes on the bumps and swerves immediately visible through their windshield.

Having watched your parents travel this road for decades, you know better than most family members the rigors and anxieties of the long, downward course. The questions you're asking have probably occurred to you (and, perhaps, were pushed away again) many times before. If you're feeling greater urgency about them now, ask yourself why. Has your mother's condition declined so much that the end is now really in sight? Her disease sounds as if it has progressed gradually. Ask her if you can confer with her neurologist about what's reasonably expectable within the next five years; perhaps the end stage is farther off than you imagine. Or is it that you feel your father's strength for tending her is now ebbing? Ask him whether his current caregiving plan is sustainable or whether you and your brothers need to step up and do more for your parents.

If your mother hasn't reached the last phases of her decline or your father hasn't reached the point of depletion, you may consider choosing to refocus on the present and be cognizant of but not dwell on their future. You wouldn't be blinding yourself to what's ahead. Rather, you'd be adaptively coping with it by decreasing your level of anxiety so you can continue to allow your parents to largely take care of themselves. If the end of their race is near, though, you and your brothers will need to initiate a dialogue among yourselves about how to help your parents accept your help. It would be best if you could work out among yourselves specific means for pitching in before presenting them to your parents. When they balk at these proposals, put the ideas aside, but keep them at the ready. If they're not deemed necessary at this point in your family's journey, they likely will be a little farther down the road.

Grandpa's Needs versus the Family's

Q: *My grandfather was recently diagnosed with terminal cancer. While his internist was extremely honest with us about there being little hope,* *he wasn't as truthful with Grandpa. Having successfully battled cancer before, my grandfather's optimistic he can do so again, and doesn't want to discuss the possibility he may not make it. My family is in turmoil because we all feel the need to talk to him about his prognosis and help him deal with the end of his life as peacefully as possible. How do we best deal with this situation for the benefit of all involved?*

A: A 2000 American Medical Association educational program entitled "End-of-Life Care" contains a section on communicating bad news that instructs physicians to assess what patients know about their conditions, ask them what they want to know, and then provide them with only as much information as they desire. If your grandfather's doctor asked him what he wanted to know and your grandfather answered, "Please don't tell me very much because I want to maintain my hope," then the physician acted in an ethical and professional manner by the standards of his profession. If the doctor failed to ask your grandfather but decided on his own how much to tell him, then the physician acted in a paternalistic and potentially harmful way and should be confronted by you and other family members.

Let's assume that the doctor did follow the AMA-suggested protocol. Your concern, then, would be with the protocol itself, because it puts the individual's needs ahead of those of family members. This is just a reflection of medicine's clinical and ethical biases to focus on the patient's disease and rights to information and treatment. "First, do no harm," consequently, may sometimes mean protecting the patient's prerogative to preserve far-fetched hope even if doing so may harm the family's need for an open dialogue. (By the same token, because of the ethical principle of medical confidentiality, you and your relatives wouldn't even know the extent of your father's condition if he hadn't given explicit permission to the physician to share that information with you.) Medical culture has changed radically in the past several decades, but, on the basic tenet that the patient is catered to first, it hasn't budged. Neither will your grandfather's physician, no matter how much you may decide to press him.

But what about your need to talk with your grandfather about his impending death? To say all the loving things you want to say to him before he dies? To make sure all his affairs are in order to avoid legal complications later on? Under ideal circumstances, all these topics would be thoroughly discussed, perhaps with the help of hospice nurses and social workers. But is a well-discussed death necessarily an "easy" death, as your question implies? I would ask you, "Easy for whom?" Perhaps for the loved ones involved but not for your grandfather. He has opted to live out the close of his life in a different way—quixotically fighting to the end. That may be the form of coping he most wants for himself. In my clinical experience, blind-eyed denial may be just as adaptive for the person facing his demise as the kind of death-bed communion we often idealize; it all depends upon the psychological makeup of the individual in the bed.

But, again, what about your needs? I'd suggest you ask your grandfather yourself whether or not he'd like to know what he's facing medically. If he says yes, then please inform him of the likelihood of his death and help him come to terms with it. But if he says no, please respect his decision by not forcing information on him. Instead, ask him, as a favor to the family, to help prepare contingency plans for any of the possible outcomes. If he should beat cancer again, then how would he want the family to help keep him healthy in the future? If he should live with cancer for a prolonged period as a chronic illness, then how would he want to be helped if he's in a disabled state? And if he should lose his battle, then how would he want the family to handle his death? By focusing on contingencies rather than prognoses, you may still wind up having the conversation you'd like while allowing your grandfather to face his final struggle in the manner he has chosen.

Getting Their House in Order

Q: *My 77-year-old dad is rapidly losing his battle with Alzheimer's. I believe it's high time he, my mother, my siblings, and I get my parents' legal and financial house in order. My mother always let my father handle these matters, and now she doesn't know what to do. I'd like to hire an attorney and perhaps a financial advisor to help guide us, but my father mistrusts the advice of outsiders and strongly dislikes lawyers. He gets angry every time I raise the subject, and my mother feels caught in the middle. I'm afraid if I go ahead and hire a legal or financial advisor, my parents will not cooperate and my dad will grow even more angry and delusional. What can I tell them and what should I do before it's too late?*

A: This is a too common and perplexing family problem that would be avoided if family members prepared last wills, advance directives, and the like long before they became ill. In trying now to tiptoe through the minefield of your family's sensitivities about money, aging, and control, there are two tactics you definitely should not use. The first is hiring a legal or financial advisor on your own. You'll only alienate your parents and siblings, who might regard what you've done as a naked power grab. The second is exerting strong pressure on your father to sign legal papers about his wishes. You'll only inflame his paranoia, a typical symptom of Alzheimer's dementia.

Instead, you'll need to do the slow, hard work of family consensus building. I'd start with your siblings. Do they share your view of the progressive, disabling nature of Dad's disease? If not, then hold a family meeting with his physician to help everyone come to a common understanding of the deteriorating medical situation. Do your siblings understand the potential legal and financial ramifications if Dad doesn't document his wishes before he is incompetent to do so? If not, a meeting with a social worker can outline the dangers, including a possible period of decreased income for your mother if your father dies and his estate winds up in probate court.

Once your siblings are in agreement with you about the need for timely action, all of you should then meet with your mother without your father present. Despite her habit of deferring to your father's prerogatives, she probably realizes his judgment is now impaired. What she needs from you is the rationale and support to make decisions for him. The most important rationale is that, by addressing legal questions now, she and your father will be in a better position to control their own lives without interference from others. Explain carefully that you and your siblings are not so concerned about your inheritance as their well-being. Appeal to her on the basis that you're worried that their well-being is in increasing jeopardy.

If your mother is now in agreement to discuss matters with your father, schedule a meeting for the entire immediate family. The focus should be on your concern for both your parents, not just your declining dad. Tell them you and your siblings would feel much better if they took steps to put their wishes in writing. Because you know how much your father detests lawyers, use the "Five Wishes" as a framework for discussion. The "Five Wishes" (available at www.agingwithdignity.org/5wishes.html) is a simple document covering medical decision making and treatments that over 4 million Americans have already used to make their preferences clear to doctors and other family members. It's a straightforward approach that meets the legal requirements of the vast majority of states in this country without containing the off-putting technical language of most legalistic documents.

My hope is that—with your show of calm, concerted support and by spreading the onus for change to both Mom and Dad—you and your siblings can at least get each of your parents to fill out the "Five Wishes" (perhaps with your help). Once the door has been opened to plan for the future, your parents may be much more likely to take the next steps and put together last wills and testaments, review their financial arrangements, and make any other necessary preparations for their demise.

If all this backfires and your father throws a fit at the very idea of a family meeting, then your mother will have undeniable evidence your father is no longer of sound-enough mind to handle their finances or other major decisions. It'll be time for her to hire a legal or financial advisor on her own to explore taking power away from him. She'll need her children's steady backing then more than ever.

Above and Beyond

Q: *My ailing mother is becoming increasingly incontinent and will soon need diapering as well as bathing. Since my father already passed away, her care has fallen on her two sons—my brother and me. I want to take care of her as best as I can, but we always were a modest family, so it's awkward and embarrassing for all of us to help her when she's naked and soiled. I can see she feels ashamed; that makes it much harder. We can't afford full-time home health aides, and it's not fair to our wives to ask them to handle this just because they're female. How can my brother and I make the situation more comfortable for Mom and for us?*

A: Incontinence is often the final straw of family caregiving. Especially incontinence of the bowels, with its need for wiping as well as diaper changing, is a backbreaker that leads many devoted family members to finally put their ill loved ones in nursing homes. It's remarkable to me that you and your brother are game for figuring out how to handle this sensitively without giving up on caring for your mom at home. There are no grand solutions to this problem, unfortunately—only an array of ideas to try:

• Too few patients and family members raise the issue of incontinence with their doctors because of embarrassment. But knowledgeable physicians, particularly urologists, have possible answers. Medications such as Detrol and anticholinergic drugs can be prescribed for the patient to cause urinary retention and/or constipation. While these drugs generally don't fully control the bowels and bladder, they regulate them to a degree, thereby allowing the patient and caregiver to make greater use of be-havioral methods (see below).

• Embarrassment also causes too few patients to agree to wear dia-pers—and too few family members to insist they do. Instead, both go along for extended periods dealing with messes that need not be as bad. It's good to hear that you, your brother, and mother already have come to grips with the necessity of Depends.

• Many hospitals and home health agencies have staff nurses who specialize in working with patients and families struggling with inconti-nence. Not only are they familiar with medications that might help, but also they can offer tailored advice on diet, environment, and behavior. For diet, a nurse may recommend that your mother avoid certain foods that are more likely to run through her gastrointestinal system or may suggest curtailing her intake of foods and liquids in the evening to avoid night accidents. For environment, the nurse may inspect your home and direct you to purchase a commode, bedpans, or other devices to give your mother the convenience to relieve herself quickly if she's lying in bed. For behavior, she may suggest that your mother sit on the toilet ev-ery 2 hours during the day, as well as twice during the night, to cut down on the number of accidents. If the initial plans she comes up with aren't foolproof, the nurse will continue to work with you and your mother to try to bring her incontinence under some control.

• If you can't afford full-time home health aides, can you pay for one for an hour or two a day? Many families hire such aides to toilet, bathe, and dress their disabled loved ones every morning to spare them-selves at least that much daily work. Most patients develop relationships with these aides (if, hopefully, the same ones come regularly) and come to accept their help with personal hygiene without humiliation. They are grateful their family members are not burdened with such hands-on care.

• If all these ideas aren't completely successful, then you'll likely need to change your mother on occasion. It sounds distasteful but has the potential for bringing the two of you into an even closer relation-ship. You and your brother should meet with your mother to discuss the predicament. Explain that you are willing to do this out of somewhat selfish reasons—you want to be able to keep her at home. Ask her if there are ways to change her that would cause her as little embarrass-ment as possible. Provide her with frequent reassurance that you aren't repulsed by doing this. Allow her to thank you profusely for helping her in this way; giving thanks may be the least she can do to maintain her dignity.

By applying all these various methods, most families, over time, learn to manage incontinence to some degree. As one of caregiving's greatest challenges, it demands the greatest imagination, delicacy, and forbearance. By assisting her with this most intimate of human functions, you and your brother will be showing her the greatest love.

Epilogue
Caregiving's Aftermath

After their brief cry in each other's embrace at their mother's graveside, the sisters quickly revert to taking care of everyone around them. They hand out tissues and put their arms around their sobbing daughters and husbands. At the gathering at the older sister's house after the burial, they circulate among the guests, exchanging news and gossip, handing out drinks, and picking up stray paper plates and napkins as they would at any other family party. It doesn't occur to them until late afternoon that, to their relatives, they seem to be holding up surprisingly well. It's not that they aren't shattered by Mom's death—they are. But each of them is in a kind of shock in which they're operating on automatic pilot, coasting through a horrific day by focusing on others.

These reactions are typical of grieving family members in the immediate aftermath of concerted caregiving. As such, they mark the beginning of a long journey of healing (after the already lengthy caregiving ordeal) in which family members often take 1–2 years to find a new sense of normalcy. While we noted previously that Kübler-Ross's stage theory of grief hasn't been supported by later research, stage theories in general still have utility as starting points for wondering about potential pathways of change as individuals and families proceed through time. In that spirit, we can follow our sisters as they go forward through the stages of their thinking about how caregiving has changed them. At times, they'll feel like newly bereft orphans; at others, like newly crowned matriarchs. Their relationship with each other and the meaning of family in their lives will also evolve.

In the early phase, lasting from a few days to 2 months, former caregivers experience a welter of feelings. Sadness predominates, but guilt runs a close second. They feel guilty because they didn't do enough. They feel guilty about feeling relieved their loved one is dead and they don't have to work so hard anymore. When they're not feeling sad or guilty, they're mostly numb—shocked to suddenly have their own lives back but unable to focus on what they're going to do. They frequently try grounding themselves in short-term work projects in the hope of avoiding being emotionally overwrought.

The sisters also attempt to use work as a refuge during this period. Details of straightening up after Mom's life occupy them for several weeks. They write notes of acknowledgment to the three dozen cousins, old neighbors, dear family friends, and former coworkers who sent flowers or condolence cards. What strikes both of them about many of the cards is that their writers describe Mom as having been "sweet." They always thought of her as more grit than sugar. This difference in perception bothers them, as if others could see something essential about their mother they couldn't. And they realize, now that she's gone, they'll never have the chance to get to know her "sweetness."

At the same time, the sisters work on disposing of Mom's possessions. She was explicit about which granddaughter should get each item of her antique china, silver platters, old handbags, scarves, jewelry, and favorite pictures and books. Organizing this complex distribution plan initially occupies the sisters' energies and distracts them from their feelings. But going back and forth to the apartment to retrieve items has an increasingly emotional effect on them. In the place's carpeting, furniture, and clothes closets is still the faint odor of Mom's cooking, perfume, and perspiration. Her essence seems to linger there. On the one hand, the scent of her is comforting to them. On the other, by making her tantalizingly present but still absent, it begins to draw their attention away from their duties to the keen sadness of their loss.

Having picked the apartment clean of its most precious items within a month of their mother's death, the sisters decide to clear it out completely and put the place up for sale. Their husbands are willing to help them remove the remaining furniture, repaint the bedroom, and steam-clean the carpets. But once this decision has been made and a plan devised, everything stalls. The emptying of the condominium apartment suddenly feels to the daughters like the erasure of their mother's life. They want Mom to endure, even in death, not disappear as quickly as it takes to cart a narrow bed and heavy couches out the door. The younger sister finds reasons to avoid going over to the apartment altogether. Even the older sister can only tolerate working there briefly before feeling overwhelmed and then departing. Cleaning out the apartment brings home a sense of finality that makes them sad and ultimately guilty. Maybe they could have done more to keep her alive longer. Perhaps they're violating her by taking apart the little world she so enjoyed. They decide that, though it makes rational sense to ready the apartment for sale, they themselves can't take part in it. Despite their husbands' pleas to work more, they beg off and finally ask Goodwill Industries to take the remaining possessions and a realtor to sell the place as quickly as possible.

After this early phase, former caregivers usually enter a longer period of grief and adjustment that can last from months to years. Immediate family members are often still full of feelings, but the support and license to express them has fallen away. The funeral-goers who mourned so fervently with them at the church and graveside have now turned back to their own lives. They not only don't want to talk about the deceased any longer but subtly recoil from family members who do. As a consequence, former caregivers frequently feel isolated and sometimes shunned. Their sadness weighs on them silently. The doubts they may have about what they did or didn't do at various junctures of their loved one's illness circle through their minds unabated. Anger wells up inside them and is suppressed. It's during this stage that former caregivers become involved in local bereavement support groups or take advantage of the grief support offered by the hospice as places where they'll feel free to express their emotions openly without inciting calls to "Please get on with your life" or, more harshly, "Stop being so negative." Through the feedback they receive at these groups, as well as by hearing the stories of other former caregivers, they frequently feel more "normal" in their grief.

This stage is also often a time when the former caregiver is challenged to redefine his or her sense of purpose. Caring for a seriously ill loved one is commonly an all-consuming affair that pulls family members away from their other meaningful roles. After the loved one's death, it isn't easy to simply return to the rhyme and reason of an earlier life. But trying to define for oneself a new life with a new sense of mission isn't easy either. Most other endeavors lack the immediacy or intensity of the high-stakes drama of caregiving. In this light, it isn't hard to understand why some former caregivers go on later to volunteer to provide care to other ill family members, as if seeking to recapture the sense of heightened importance they felt while on the front lines.

In this middle phase, the older sister struggles in several ways. She misses her mother terribly. When her husband is at work or in the basement, the house now feels uncomfortably deserted to her. When she awakens in the morning, she still finds herself thinking about what to make Mom for breakfast before catching and chiding herself. Because she isn't inclined to dwell on sadness, her thoughts run quickly in other directions. She feels guilt periodically that she didn't do more to convince the mother to choose to fight longer. But she assigns greater blame to her sister, whom she believes practically encouraged Mom to die. As a consequence, she finds herself shying away from calling or seeing her younger sibling. The older sister's daughters, meanwhile, keep asking her out to lunch and to see her grandchildren. But the older sister is often out of sorts and never seems to feel fully present when with them. She returns to work at the bank but feels as though she's just going through the motions there as well. Even when her husband takes her on a vacation to the Caribbean to reinvigorate their marriage, she appreciates the effort but comes home still feeling empty and restless and unsure of what to do with herself.

During this stage, the younger sister experiences different difficulties. She, too, misses Mom but, because she didn't live with her, not as an integral part of her daily life. What she misses instead are her toughness and firm support—the qualities the younger sister could now use to better handle Mom's death. Unfortunately, even clear memories of the mother's strengths are not available to her during this time. As little as she likes to recall the scene, the younger sister finds her thoughts suffused with visual images of her mother, looking unnaturally pale and waxen, with her head pressed against the railing of her hospital bed near the end of her life. However forcefully she tries to push these images away, they play out in her head like a repeating video loop she can't turn off. The terrible scene distracts her attention while she's back at work. It preoccupies her while eating dinner with her husband. It's only when she reluctantly goes back into psychotherapy for the first time in many years that she discovers she's suffering from a form of posttraumatic stress disorder and begins to learn skills to wrest back her mind. She even goes on psychiatric medicine for 6 months to reduce the intensity of her traumatic memories and the anxiety they provoke.

During the last stage, which commonly occurs between 6 months and 2 years after the patient's demise, there's some resolution of the shock and hard feelings of the earlier phases. If time itself doesn't actually heal, then the flow of daily living tends to carry people along familiar byways but also ultimately into new currents and uncharted waters whose challenges demand attention to the present, not the past. The sadness over the loved one's death is still evident, but its intensity lessens as rationalization sets in: At least she's no longer suffering and merely existing, caregivers are apt to say. Anger, largely a byproduct of the sadness, slowly fizzles. Guilt comes and goes but eventually is reduced by the realization that the disease took its own unerring course and God may have had His own unswerving plan. The past does still matter; the ordeal of caregiving remains painful in their memories; the loved one's loss is still foremost in their minds. But the emphasis gradually shifts from dwelling on the pain and loss to deriving wisdom from the caregiving and end-of-life experiences to cherish the family more, savor living more, and count their blessings with more intention and awareness.

An essential part of making this shift during this stage is for caregivers to develop new purposeful activities. For some, this may mean taking up hobbies during time previously devoted to giving care. Some create testaments to the lessons of their loved ones' lives. For example, they may tend a garden their deceased relative planted. Or they may volunteer in a local school where their loved one taught. Or, in a more symbolic gesture, they may take charge of candle lighting at their churches as a way of keeping alive the spark their family member had let shine in the world.

Others devise or participate in projects commemorating their loved ones' struggles with serious illness. They may walk in annual marches to cure Alzheimer's dementia, diabetes, or cancer. They may set up neighborhood fund-raising luncheons or educational programs. Or they may volunteer at county senior centers to deliver Meals on Wheels to other homebound ill people.

Yet other former caregivers will seek activities that support family caregiving itself. They may become political advocates for federal and state government programs to allocate funding for respite care for weary caregivers. They may continue attending caregiver support groups, acting as mentors for family members who are encountering the rigors of taking care of a seriously ill loved one for the first time. Or they may keep their hands in caregiving proper, helping out relatives, friends, and neighbors with arduous duties, whether or not they received such aid during their own caregiving tenures.

Regardless of which activity a former caregiver chooses, if it's a meaningful distillation to her of her own family's experience, then it will help transform the ordeal and loss to something more. A new purposeful endeavor won't remove the sting of death but is often a salve to its pain. It will allow a former caregiver to continue caring and growing by integrating what she's been through into new goals she'll work toward during the rest of her life.

At the outset of this last stage, the older sister is still floundering. Her job and marriage don't fill the void she feels. She rejects her husband's suggestion that she take up tennis; she doesn't much feel like doing anything. It's only when an older gentleman who lives down the block falls and breaks a hip that she begins to stir. A widower who was married to a woman with whom Mom regularly played canasta years ago, the older sister has known him slightly since she was a girl. At first she merely does what any good neighbor would do, dropping off covered dishes with dinner several times after he returns from the hospital following hip surgery. But because she notices his house is a shambles—lacking proper housekeeping and repairs because of his wife's absence and his recent infirmities—the older sister soon makes herself indispensable. She pins up her hair, brings over her vacuum cleaner, and scrubs every mismatched plate in the house. Without even asking his permission, she buys cans of white and blue paint and sets to stripping wallpaper and repainting the kitchen. She makes her husband bring over his toolkit to fix the front door lock and replace a broken window pane in the bathroom. The widower, of course, is grateful and elated. When she reflects on it, the older sister finds that, for the first time in a while, she's pleased.

It doesn't come as a complete shock to her but as a reminder of something that slipped her mind for a time: The older sister knows she needs to be needed. This insight prompts her to step back and reassess things. Is working and making her husband dinner really the way she wants to spend her life? Probably not, she admits. She needs people and projects and causes; she's most fulfilled when most accomplished and acknowledged. The older sister knows that, if she were here, Mom would push her to change. And so the older sister makes some decisions: She cuts back her hours at the bank and starts baby-sitting her youngest grandchildren 2 days a week. She continues checking on the widower almost nightly. And she begins to run errands and do chores for some of the other older people on her street.

She continues to miss her mother every day. She still occasionally calls out to her from the bottom of the staircase before remembering her mother is gone. But when she's taking care of others, the older sister feels that Mom's presence is nearly palpable. Her determination continues to animate the daughter's life. It isn't as much fun as having lunch together, the older sister cracks, but as remedy for grief it'll have to suffice.

Her younger sibling, during this time, still struggles to an extent. The images of her dying mother continue to pop into her consciousness without warning but lack the vividness they had previously. At the same time, she's been able to bring more clearly to mind earlier memories of her mother as a vital, commanding woman—sometimes too commanding, as the younger sister now recalls. The goal, says the psychotherapist with whom she continues to meet weekly, is to achieve a balance between sadness and appreciation—to be able to sort among her recollections of various times in her mother's life without getting stuck on only the most painful, final moments. Having made some progress, she believes she can go further toward remembering her mother realistically within the context of a lifetime's joys and strivings.

But as the power of the deathbed images begins to fade, the guilt that accompanies them remains. Part of her knows she did what was humane—giving her mother permission to stop fighting and therefore die more peacefully. But another part of her wonders if she were just trying to end the ordeal sooner to better spare herself. This fear is fueled by her older sister's obvious avoidance of her nowadays. Despite reassurances from her daughters and even her eldest niece that she did the right thing, the younger sister finds that her sibling's cool reception incites her guilt nonetheless. She has lost her mother; she has no intention of losing her older sibling, too. So, the younger sister calls her and confronts her. Don't take your sadness out on me by blaming me for contributing to Mom's death, the younger sister says. Don't push me away because I supported Mom's decision against your arguments. The conversation produces a partial success. The older sister admits to feelings of hurt and anger she knows she's directing at her sibling. She'll try to stop, she promises, but believes she's entitled to feel the way she does. The sisters agree to disagree on the issue and to spend more time together to attempt to sort out their differences.

Even after this exchange, the younger sister has nagging self-doubts about the role she played. Coincidentally, she receives a call from her mother's hospice nurse doing routine follow-up to see how the family members are coping. Though she at first responds that all are well, the younger sister soon mentions she feels guilty for supporting Mom's decision. The nurse listens and then relates that many family members react similarly, but what's important is respecting the patient's right to choose. Having already heard such advice, the younger sister thanks her politely and prepares to hang up. But then the nurse surprises her by asking her whether she'd like to talk further with patients and their relatives about this issue by becoming a hospice volunteer.

It seems such an unlikely idea. Prone to depression and already contending with images of one dying person, why would she want to expose herself to more? She discusses the prospect with her therapist, who thinks it entails the risk of increasing her symptoms but also, paradoxically, could help rid her of doubts by putting her in a position to empathize with other caregivers. Her husband suggests she at least try it.

At first, it doesn't go well. Sitting in strange bedrooms and chatting with two different hospice patients—an elderly woman dying of emphysema and a middle-aged man failing from colon cancer—initially intensifies her feelings about her mother. She has frightening nightmares in which Mom suffers terribly and she watches helplessly behind a glass wall. But, after sticking with the volunteer work anyway, the dreams subside as she gets to know the people whom she's helping. The woman is very gentle and soft-spoken. Her daughter is around the younger sister's age and feels a mix of love, discouragement, and guilt, as she did. The man's wife is very assertive, like Mom. Even facing the patients' deaths with them doesn't tip the younger sister into depression. On the contrary, she seems to have a steadiness—some might say toughness—that helps anchor these families with whom she's sharing the end of life. Perhaps after fighting depression for so many years, the younger sister has developed a talent for managing sadness. It's a talent that may lack the spitfire energy of her mother and older sister. But it shares with them a kind of dogged determination to help her and others get through the worst of times.

Two years after the mother's death, the sisters derive similar lessons from the experiences of caregiving and watching a parent die. They both dreadfully fear getting cancer. They each have completed living wills to make their wishes known in the event they're incapacitated. They both have purchased long-term care insurance policies so that, if the time should come, they can go into nursing homes rather than have their children take care of them the way they took care of their parents. Each of them talks out loud to Mom every day and visits her grave often, telling her about the doings in their lives and how much they wish she were there to join them.

And yet, like any two independent and dissimilar siblings, they think and feel quite differently. Having gained the confidence she can endure from her volunteer hospice work, the younger sister gives it up after a year. She concentrates her energies, instead, on caring for her grandchildren—exactly what she'd planned to do before Mother became sick. The older sister, in contrast, has expanded her involvement with the neighborhood's senior citizens. What started as a favor—feeding a hobbled old man—escalates into a mission of organizing church volunteers to provide repairs, food, and companionship for dozens of elder congregants on an ongoing basis. The younger sister talks openly with her daughters about getting older and about how she intends not to burden them with her care. Despite buying the long-term care insurance, the older sister hints to her daughters that she expects them to want to take care of her in the future. (After all, she gladly did it for her parents and is doing it for other people's parents. She believes she's consequently entitled to it from her children one day.)

A fundamental change has happened to the family as a whole since the death of their matriarch. More so than any of them realized during her lifetime, Mom was the linchpin to all family interactions. When, during the first Thanksgiving after Mom's death, several of the married granddaughters go to their in-laws for turkey rather than attending the family's gathering as usual, it dawns on everyone the family no longer coheres in the same way. This marks the advent of another loss. Cousins who were always close under the watchful eye of their common grandmother are beginning to drift away from one another in her absence. The cousins' children—the generation of great-grandchildren—will never get the chance to get to know one another by carousing at overflowing holiday events as their parents did.

But there's a certain freedom in this, too. Without Mom's dominating presence, the sisters feel like they're growing into the roles of matriarchs for their respective broods. They now each get to call the shots when planning family dinners and sit at the heads of their own crowded tables. In truth, their mother's demise means they no longer see each other as much either. Yet, the bond between them is still strong. They are their parents' children; no one else in the world shares as much. They were their parents' caregivers; they worked side by side to give them love and cherish the time they had together.

Resources

In one respect, family caregivers are fortunate there's an abundance of available resources to help guide them through a prolonged medical crisis. On the Internet, especially, the number of outlets devoted to providing information to caregivers—on everything from talking with doctors to demystifying the intricacies of health insurance to coping emotionally—has increased substantially since the beginning of this century. Online psychological support is also offered widely. Some of this takes the form of fostering "connectivity"—putting caregivers of similar backgrounds in touch with one another (either virtually through chat rooms or in real life) to increase opportunities for swapping ideas, commiserating, and even mentoring.

In another respect, however, the sheer quantity of information sources for caregivers has produced what many will regard as a dizzying, stupefying array. There are multiple advocacy groups that appear to cover the same waterfront. There are overlapping governmental institutions and programs, a plethora of bureaucracies and initiatives. There are so many sources of medical knowledge that it's difficult to determine which are authoritative and which more suspect.

So that you can avail yourself of the resources pertinent to you and your family, a list of the most respected websites, organizations, and publications follows. First, though, you should consider a few strategies for proceeding as effectively as possible:

• *Get the lay of the land.* To prepare yourself for caregiving, you'll need to know the potential courses of your loved one's illness. That means learning about medical conditions about which you may have scant knowledge. The more you learn, of course, the more you'll figure out what else you need to know. It's best, then, to start out with basic information about the disease (for example, its typical causes and effects) before moving on to more sophisticated considerations (for instance, comparing side-effect profiles of different medication regimens or learning about the latest research studies). In most cases, therefore, it's wise to go to general medical and health websites (see below) to learn about a condition in order to get the lay of the land before turning to the more comprehensive and consequently complex information available from disease-specific organizations.

• *Search globally, find locally* . . . In our Internet-connected world, it's not unusual to be able to find national and international resources for caregiving more easily than you can local ones. But it's probably local resources that will make the greatest difference to you and your family for coping over time. Most websites for national organizations can steer you to local support groups and individuals, local home healthcare agencies, or local caregiver support programs. Be sure to click on the state listings or put in your zip code (if the site offers these features) to find the resources closest to your home.

• . . . *But search locally, too.* Most towns and counties have their own websites that list social service agencies in your community. The blue pages in your local phone book probably list the same resources. Your local Area Agency on Aging (see below under "Other Resources") can offer suggestions for caring for an elderly family member. Contact them and inquire about caregiver support services, home health aides, respite care, Meals on Wheels programs, and the like. If they don't have the information you need, they likely will be able to direct you to the right agency to call.

• *Seek connections as well as information.* The people from whom you'll garner the greatest knowledge and support are likely those who have been or are going through similar caregiving experiences. Take advantage of all opportunities offered to meet others and talk shop. If you don't have the time to do this in person by attending support groups, use the Internet and phone calls to reach out. You will feel less alone.

GENERAL MEDICAL AND HEALTH WEBSITES

familydoctor.org

Created by the American Academy of Family Practice to educate non-professionals, this website provides basic reliable information, written in clear, simple language, about a broad range of health issues affecting adults and kids. It's a good place to start learning about any medical or psychosocial problem.

ThirdAge (www.thirdage.com)

This website has materials on health, relationships, money, and work, as well as myriad links to other sites on seniors, nursing and rehab, Alzheimer's dementia, and other health conditions.

Healthfinder (www.healthfinder.gov)

Selected as one of the 10 most useful websites by the Medical Library Association, this is the Internet portal for the National Health Information Center of the U.S. Department of Health and Human Services. It draws on disease and health promotion information from governmental agencies and over 1,500 health-related organizations.

HealthWeb (www.healthweb.org)

This is a search portal run by health sciences libraries of the National Network of Libraries of Medicine and the Committee for Institutional Cooperation. It links to sites on topics ranging from AIDS, allied health, and alternative medicine to transplantation, urology, and women's health.

DISEASE-SPECIFIC ORGANIZATIONS AND WEBSITES

Alzheimer's Dementia

Alzheimer's Association
225 North Michigan Ave., Fl. 17
Chicago, IL 60601
Website: www.alz.org
Phone: 1-800-272-3900

This organization offers basic and cutting-edge information, sponsors advocacy activities such as its Memory Walks, and runs local support groups and family caregiver trainings. Its website contains advice for caregivers on working with physicians, making legal decisions, and managing a loved one's behavior.

ALZwell Caregiver Support
Prism Innovations, Inc.
50 Amuxen Court
Islip, NY 11751
Website: www.alzwell.com

This website, along with Prism's ElderCare Online (www.ec-online.net), is intended to provide resources and support for family caregivers coping with Alzheimer's and other issues generally associated with aging. It has chat rooms and bulletin boards, offers tips and suggestions, and sells a 20-page handbook on coping with the various stages of Alzheimer's.

Alzheimer's Disease Education and Referral Center (ADEAR)
P.O. Box 8250
Silver Spring, MD 20907-8250
Website: www.alzheimers.org
Phone: 1-800-438-4380

A service of the National Institute on Aging, the center has a staff of information specialists to answer your questions, offers free publications on the disease, and makes referrals to local support services and specialized medical centers. It also publishes *Connections,* a newsletter for health professionals.

Brain Injury

Tbi-help.org (www.tbi-help.org)

Developed by the Jamaica (New York) Hospital Medical Center with a grant from the United Hospital Fund of New York, this search portal provides links to websites on the medical details and legal ramifications of traumatic brain injuries.

Cancer

American Cancer Society
Website: www.cancer.org
Phone: 1-800-ACS-2345

With 3,400 local offices, this Atlanta-based organization has a strong community presence for providing information, sponsoring support groups, and connecting cancer survivors of similar backgrounds. Its website contains extensive information for caregivers about treatment decision making and coping.

National Cancer Institute
National Institutes of Health
9000 Bethesda Pike
Bethesda, MD 20892
Website: www.cancer.gov
Phone: 1-800-4-CANCER (1-800-422-6237)

The primary agency for cancer research in the United States, it offers free fact sheets, publications, and up-to-date news and resources on all types of cancer. It also lists information on clinical trials around the nation. You can call or chat online with an information specialist.

National Coalition for Cancer Survivorship
1010 Wayne Avenue, Suite 770
Silver Spring, MD 20910
Website: www.cansearch.org
Phone: 1-877-NCCS-YES (1-877-622-7937)

This organization seeks to empower cancer survivors by offering information on every type of cancer and many aspects of cancer care, listing noted cancer centers, and fostering peer networking. Its Cancer Survival Toolbox is a free 10-part audio program to help survivors and caregivers meet the challenges of cancer.

Association of Cancer Online Resources (www.acor.org)

This website serves as a host for online discussion groups, mailing lists, and other websites on many kinds of cancer, including rare types, for both patients and caregivers. This is a superb resource for connecting with others.

OncoLink
Abramson Cancer Center of the University of Pennsylvania
3400 Spruce Street, 2 Donner
Philadelphia, PA 19104-4283
Website: www.oncolink.com

This is an excellent information source on the latest scientific advances in the treatments of a wide array of cancers.

Heart Disease

American Heart Association
7272 Greenville Avenue
Dallas, TX 75231
Website: www.americanheart.org
Phone: 1-800-AHA-USA-1 (1-800-242-8721)

This organization provides information on heart disease and stroke, as well as tips on leading a healthier lifestyle. Its website lists local chapters and resources. It also contains information on emergency cardiovascular care and CPR.

Mental Health Issues

NAMI (National Alliance on Mental Illness)
Colonial Place Three
2107 Wilson Boulevard, Suite 300
Arlington, VA 22201-3042
Website: www.nami.org
Phone: 1-800-950-NAMI (1-800-950-6264)

This is a self-help support and advocacy organization for patients and their family members contending with major psychiatric illnesses, including bipolar disorder, severe depression, and anxiety. It has over 1,000 local affiliates that sponsor support and advocacy groups. Its Information Helpline (above) can provide referrals to local resources.

Multiple Sclerosis

National Multiple Sclerosis Society
733 Third Avenue
New York, NY 10017
Website: www.nationalmssociety.org
Phone: 1-800-FIGHT-MS (1-800-344-4867)

This organization supports research, provides education to patients, caregivers, and professionals (including online webcasts), and sponsors local support groups throughout the country.

Parkinson's Disease

National Parkinson Foundation
1501 NW 9th Avenue / Bob Hope Road
Miami, FL 33136-1494
Website: www.parkinson.org
Phone: 1-800-327-4545

Through its efforts to promote research, education, and support, the foundation aims to improve the lives of patients and their family caregivers. It identifies qualified medical practices around the country as Care Centers.

Stroke

National Stroke Association
9707 East Easter Lane
Englewood, CO 80112
Website: www.stroke.org
Phone: 1-800-STROKES (1-800-787-6537)

This advocacy organization publishes *Stroke Smart* magazine and directs patients and family members to regional resources. It has produced stroke prevention guidelines for those who've already had a stroke to share with their doctors in order to prevent additional strokes.

For all other diseases:

The American Self-Help Group Clearinghouse (www.selfhelpgroups.org; 973-326-6789) can direct you to support groups on common and rare diseases.

CAREGIVING RESOURCES

Age Concern New Zealand
Level 4, West Block, Education House
178 Willis Street
Wellington, New Zealand
Website: www.ageconcern.org.nz
Phone: +64 (0)4 801 9338

This organization is a federation of New Zealand local councils that provide information, resources, and services to facilitate the well-being of older people and their loved ones. Its website highlights its "Ageing is Living" project, which promotes a positive view of getting older.

CAPS (Children of Aging Parents)
P.O. Box 167
Richboro, PA 18954
Wewbsite: www.caps4caregivers.org
Phone: 1-800-227-7294

With support groups in Pennsylvania, New Jersey, California, and other states, as well as an online support group, this national organization primarily promotes communication among caregiving adult children. Its quarterly newsletter publishes articles on such topics as elder law, avoiding burnout, and getting along with professionals.

Caregiver Media Group
Website: www.caregiver.com
Phone: 1-800-829-2734

Publisher of *Today's Caregiver* magazine and organizer of regional Fearless Caregiver Conferences, this media company is a leading purveyor of practical information about caregiving. Its website has online discussion groups and chat rooms.

Caregiver Network, Inc.
2 Oaklawn Gardens, Unit C
Toronto, Ontario M4V2C6, Canada
Website: www.caregiver.on.ca
Phone: 416-323-1090

This Canadian organization focuses on providing information about caring for an aging family member. It publishes a quarterly newsletter and has produced a 13-part TV/video series on caregiving.

Carers Australia
P.O. Box 73
Deakin West ACT 2600
Unit 2, 43-49 Geils Court, Deakin 2600, Australia
Website: www.carersaustralia.com.au
Phone: +61 (0)2 6122 9900

The national voice of carers in Australia, this organization offers information on research, policy, and advocacy, as well as listings of Carer Associations and Commonwealth Carer Resource Centres in states throughout the country.

Carers New Zealand
Freepost 3739
Mangonui, Far North 0557, New Zealand
Website: www.carers.net.nz
Phone: +64 (0)9 406 0412

Members of this organization receive its magazine, *Caring Times*, and other publications and resources. Its website offers online communities, a resource library, and carer classifieds, as well as a local service locator.

Carers UK (Carers National Association)
20-25 Glasshouse Yard
London EC1A 4JT, United Kingdom
Website: www.carersuk.org.uk
Phone: 020 7490 8818

The United Kingdom's leading organization of carers, it has 110 branches throughout England, Wales, Scotland, and Northern Ireland. Its free Carers-Line and Carers Online provide advice and information. It also sponsors specialized services for young carers and for carers who are still working.

Crossroads Association
10 Regent Place
Rugby Warwickshire CV21 2PN, United Kingdom
Website: www.crossroads.org.uk
Phone: +44 (0)845 450 0350

This charitable English organization sends out trained Carer Support Workers to carers' homes for visits and to provide short respites. Its website lists the availability of local services.

FamilyCareAmerica (www.familycareamerica.com)
Created by entrepreneur Ron Moore, founder of Office America and CarMax, this website provides information on emotional issues, housing, legal matters, care facilities, money, medical care, and transportation, among other issues.

Family Caregiver Alliance
180 Montgomery Street, Suite 1100
San Francisco, CA 94104
Website: www.caregiver.org
Phone: 1-800-445-8106

After serving as the lead agency in California's statewide system of Caregiver Resource Centers, this organization established the National Center on Caregiving to promote caregiver support programs and policies in every state in the country. Its website offers numerous fact sheets and handbooks, best-practice models for caregiver education and support programs, and access to electronic newsletters and online discussion groups. Its information specialists can direct you to resources in your community.

National Alliance for Caregiving
4720 Montgomery Lane, 5th Floor
Bethesda, MD 20814
Website: www.caregiving.org
Phone: 301-718-8444

A joint coalition of nearly 40 organizations focusing on family caregiving, the alliance conducts research, does policy analysis, and promotes public awareness of caregivers' concerns. Its website offers caregiving tips and publications on hospital discharge planning, palliative care, and aging parents. It also has reviews with ratings on over 1,000 books, videotapes, and other materials on caregiving.

National Family Caregivers Association
10400 Connecticut Avenue, Suite 500
Kensington, MD 20895-3944
Website: www.thefamilycaregiver.org
Phone: 1-800-896-3650

The leading organization in the United States supporting family caregivers offers education, support, and advocacy. Its website provides caregiving tips and information, including extensive materials on communicating effectively with healthcare professionals, as well as access to dozens of narratives of caregivers' personal stories. Its quarterly newsletter is filled with pragmatic suggestions for typical caregiver concerns.

Net of Care
Beth Israel Medical Center
Department of Pain Medicine and Palliative Care
The Family Caregiver Program
First Avenue at 16th Street
New York, NY 10003
Website: www.netofcare.org

This website contains the Caregiver Resource Directory, a well-organized, comprehensive guide to dealing with the healthcare system, managing common patient symptoms, and attending to your own emotional, physical, and spiritual needs. Its online newsletter answers frequently asked questions with clear, practical advice.

Rosalynn Carter Institute for Caregiving
Georgia Southwestern State University
Americus, GA 31709
Website: www.rci.gsw.edu

The institute forms partnerships with companies and professional organizations to conduct research, advance pro-caregiver public policies, and identify and award best caregiving support programs. Its website offers publications on caregiving tips and publishes moving articles by Shirley Loflin, a current family caregiver.

The Well Spouse Association
63 West Main Street, Suite H
Freehold, NJ 07728
Website: www.wellspouse.org
Phone: 1-800-838-0879

Inspired by the book *Mainstay* by Maggie Strong (see next section), this organization is dedicated to supporting the spouses and partners of the chronically ill and disabled. It has support groups throughout the country and sponsors respites and conferences. Its bimonthly newsletter frequently publishes first-person accounts of spousal caregivers.

Notable Books on Family Caregiving

Always on Call: When Illness Turns Families into Caregivers (2004), edited by Carol Levine. A United Hospital Fund Book published by Vanderbilt University Press.

American Medical Association Guide to Home Caregiving (2001) by the American Medical Association. Published by John Wiley & Sons.

Caregiving: The Spiritual Journey of Love, Loss, and Renewal (1999) by Beth Witrogen McLeod. Published by John Wiley & Sons.

Caregiving and Loss: Family Needs, Professional Responses (2001), edited by Kenneth J. Doka & Joyce D. Davidson. Published by Hospice Foundation of America.

The Fearless Caregiver: How to Get the Best Care for Your Loved One and Still Have a Life of Your Own (2001) by Gary Barg. Published by Capital Books.

Love, Honor, & Value: A Family Caregiver Speaks Out about the Choices & Challenges of Caregiving (2002) by Suzanne Geffen Mintz. Published by Capital Books.

Mainstay: For the Well Spouse of the Chronically Ill (1997) by Maggie Strong. Published by Bradford Books.

The 36-Hour Day: A Family Guide to Caring for Persons with Alzheimer's Disease, Related Dementing Illnesses, and Memory Loss Later in Life (1999) by Nancy L. Mace and Peter V. Rabins. Published by Johns Hopkins University Press.

END-OF-LIFE RESOURCES

Americans for Better Care of the Dying
1700 Diagonal Road, Suite 635
Alexandria, VA 22314
Website: www.abcd-caring.org

This organization primarily works toward public policy changes to improve end-of-life care. But its website contains its *Handbook for Mortals*, an end-of-life guide that has sections on living with illness, finding meaning, helping caregivers, talking with your doctor, and many other topics.

Hospice Foundation of America
1621 Connecticut Avenue NW, Suite 300
Washington, DC 20009
Website: www.hospicefoundation.org
Phone: 1-800-854-3402

The goal of this organization is to enhance the role of hospices in the American healthcare system. It holds an annual teleconference on various topics in hospice care that is seen by 125,000 viewers in venues around the country. Its website contains numerous articles on dealing with loss and grief, as well as the Meuser and Marwit Caregiving Assessment Tool, the American Medical Association's Caregiver Self-Assessment Questionnaire, and the U.S. Administration on Aging's Caregiver Survival Tips.

National Hospice and Palliative Care Organization
1700 Diagonal Road, Suite 625
Alexandria, VA 22314
Website: www.nhpco.org
Phone: 703-837-1500

The largest membership organization for American hospice programs, it offers general information on hospice and palliative care. Through its website, it can direct you to local providers of such services.

FAITH-BASED RESOURCES

Faith in Action
Website: www.fiavolunteers.org
Phone: 877-324-8411

A program of the Robert Wood Johnson Foundation that's active in nearly 50 states, Faith in Action brings together volunteers from many faiths to care for neighbors with long-term health needs. Volunteers typically pick up groceries, provide rides to the doctor, and visit. The program's website can tell you which local initiatives are close to your home.

Rest Ministries
P.O. Box 502928
San Diego, CA 92150
Website: www.restministries.org
Phone: 1-888-751-REST (1-888-751-7378)

This is a Christian organization devoted to serving people who live with chronic illness or pain and their families. It publishes *HopeKeepers Magazine* and sponsors Hopekeepers support groups around the country. Through its website, you can access articles, a chat room, and free daily devotionals.

OTHER RESOURCES

American Association of Homes and Services for the Aging
2519 Connecticut Avenue NW
Washington, DC 20008
Website: www.aahsa.org
Phone: 202-783-2242

Members of this organization represent most of the nursing homes and assisted-living facilities in the United States. Through its website, you can get general information about choosing a facility for your loved one, including listings of homes and services in your area. A section on caregiving describes how to talk with a family member about going into a nursing home and how to make the transition to a new living arrangement go smoothly.

ARCH National Respite Network
800 Eastowne Drive, Suite 105
Chapel Hill, NC 27514
Website: www.archrespite.org
Phone: 919-490-5577

This organization's website offers basic information about various types of respite care—temporary relief for caregivers from caring for an ill or disabled loved one. Its Respite Locator Service is a listing of respite services with contact information in your city or state.

Friends' Health Connection
P.O. Box 114
New Brunswick, NJ 08903
Website: www.friendshealthconnection.org
Phone: 1-800-48-FRIEND (1-800-483-7436)

This organization's mission is to connect people who have had similar experiences with illness for mutual support. That includes family caregivers of similar backgrounds and experiences. Participants communicate via e-mail, letters, and telephone to share wisdom gained and to provide comfort and encouragement to one another.

National Association for Home Care & Hospice
228 Seventh Street, SE
Washington, DC 20003
Website: www.nahc.org
Phone: 202-547-7424

The website for this trade organization has the useful guide *How to Choose a Home Care Provider*, which contains sections on types of services, how to pay for them, and how to choose the right provider for your loved one. An online bookstore sells the booklets "Home Care Bill of Rights," "Hospice Patient's Bill of Rights," and other titles on home care and hospice.

National Association of Area Agencies on Aging
1730 Rhode Island Avenue NW, Suite 1200
Washington, DC 20036
Website: www.n4a.org
Phone: 202-872-0888

This is the umbrella organization for this country's 655 area agencies on aging (AAAs) and 230 Title VI Native American aging programs. The AAAs and Title VI programs provide local links for a broad range of services for eligible older adults and their caregivers, including care management, assistance with transportation and housing, senior centers, adult day care programs, Meals on Wheels programs, caregiver support initiatives, and many others. Its Eldercare Locator to help you find the AAA or Title VI program in your area is available through its website or by calling 1-800-677-1116.

National Association of Professional Geriatric Care Managers
1604 North Country Club Road
Tucson, AZ 85716-3102
Website: www.caremanager.org
Phone: 520-881-8008

As the website for this organization explains, a geriatric care manager is a social worker, nurse, gerontologist, or psychologist who works privately with older adults and their families to create effective plans of care. The website has listings of geriatric care managers in your area as well as Internet links to other websites on services for older adults, caregiving, and medical information.

Index